An Atlas of Investigation and Therapy

# INTERVENTIONAL CARDIOLOGY

# An Atlas of Investigation and Therapy

# INTERVENTIONAL CARDIOLOGY

## Bernhard Meier, MD

Professor and Chairman of Cardiology
Swiss Cardiovascular Center Bern
University Hospital
Bern, Switzerland

**CLINICAL PUBLISHING**

OXFORD

Distributed worldwide by
CRC Press
Boca Raton    London    New York    Washington D.C.

**Clinical Publishing**
An imprint of Atlas Medical Publishing Ltd
Oxford Centre for Innovation
Mill Street, Oxford OX2 0JX, UK

Tel: +44 1865 811116
Fax: +44 1865 251550
Web: www.clinicalpublishing.co.uk

Distributed by:

CRC Press LLC
2000 NW Corporate Blvd
Boca Raton, FL 33431, USA
E-mail: orders@crcpress.com

CRC Press UK
23—25 Blades Court
Deodar Road
London SW15 2NU, UK
E-mail: crcpress@itps.co.uk

© Atlas Medical Publishing Ltd 2004

First published 2004

A catalogue record for this book is available from the British Library

ISBN 1 904392 11 3

**The publisher makes no representation, express or implied, that the dosages in
this book are correct. Readers must therefore always check the product
information and clinical procedures with the most up-to-date published product
information and data sheets provided by the manufacturers and the most recent
codes of conduct and safety regulations. The authors and the publisher do not
accept any liability for any errors in the text or for the misuse or misapplication of
material in this work.**

Printed in Spain by Fisa - Escudo de Oro, S A. Barcelona

# Contents

# Contributors

*Francesca Como*, MD
Cardiology
Swiss Cardiovascular Center Bern
University Hospital
Bern, Switzerland

*Etienne Delacrétaz*, MD
Professor of Cardiology
Swiss Cardiovascular Center Bern
University Hospital
Bern, Switzerland

*Jürg Fuhrer*, MD
Director of Rhythmology
Swiss Cardiovascular Center Bern
University Hospital
Bern, Switzerland

*Otto Hess*, MD
Professor and Co-Chairman of Cardiology
Swiss Cardiovascular Center Bern
University Hospital
Bern, Switzerland

*Bernhard Meier*, MD
Professor and Chairman of Cardiology
Swiss Cardiovascular Center Bern
University Hospital
Bern, Switzerland

*Markus Schwerzmann*, MD
Cardiology
Swiss Cardiovascular Center Bern
University Hospital
Bern, Switzerland

*Nicola Schwick*, MD
Cardiology
Swiss Cardiovascular Center Bern
University Hospital
Bern, Switzerland

*Christian Seiler*, MD, FACC, FESC
Professor of Cardiology
Director of Echocardiography
Swiss Cardiovascular Center Bern
University Hospital
Bern, Switzerland

*Mario Togni*, MD
Cardiology
Swiss Cardiovascular Center Bern
University Hospital
Bern, Switzerland

*Sandy Watson*, RN, BN
Cardiology
Swiss Cardiovascular Center Bern
University Hospital
Bern, Switzerland

*Stephan Windecker*, MD
Director of Invasive Cardiology
Swiss Cardiovascular Center Bern
University Hospital
Bern, Switzerland

*Thomas Wolber*, MD
Cardiology
Swiss Cardiovascular Center Bern
University Hospital
Bern, Switzerland

# Preface

This Atlas presents a selection of topics in diagnostic and interventional cardiology. It appears too voluminous at first to be read from A to Z, although it is far from being a comprehensive review of the topic. It is a sampler of pertinent pieces of knowledge, tidbits, tricks, and knacks, and helpful advice for people involved in interventional cardiology or often in contact with it, and reminds the reader of the fact that interventional cardiology does not stop at coronary interventions. The Atlas is not unlike a Sunday newspaper: you may pick up the paper after lunch on Sunday and before you know it, it is suppertime; you will not have learned everything; you will not have read everything; you will not have understood everything, and you will certainly not have memorized everything. But you will have gathered a lot of new and interesting information and you will have had an entertaining afternoon. This is exactly what this book is supposed to do for you.

The Atlas starts with a warm-up exercise for your brain cells. The physiology of coronary collateral circulation is explained with just enough depth to lift the reader above the crowd when it comes to understanding the enigmatic but often life-saving role of coronary collaterals. The subsequent chapter on frugal coronary angioplasty opens a different view on one of the most common interventions in modern medicine. The view deviates from evidence- or safety-driven exhaustive employment of options and techniques. It shows a way to get to the finish line swiftly, economically, and with less ado. Alcohol ablation of septal hypertrophy is a 'new kid on the block' of interventional cardiology. The criteria for patients qualifying for the procedure are described and only a few specialists are needed for this intervention. Nevertheless, the modern cardiologist must know what it is about, how it is done, and what one can expect from it.

A much more common feature is a patent foramen ovale. One of four human beings walks around with one. It comes to the attention of the physician when paradoxical emboli occur, migraine becomes intolerable, or a diving career is jeopardized. The pertinent chapter draws on the expertise of a centre with extensive experience in this domain and puts this topic well into perspective. After all, this already is the second most common intervention in many a catheterization laboratory and will be just that in all before long.

A chapter presents the method for exclusion of the left atrial appendage to obviate the need for anticoagulation in atrial fibrillation. It is unknown whether this method will be commonplace in some years or whether it will be relegated to the medical museum. Three different devices are on the market for it but they are challenged by new and more simple ways of anticoagulation as the procedure is by no means as trivial as the closure of a patent foramen ovale.

Electrophysiology is the topic of the next two chapters. First, ablation of various forms of tachycardia is described, beautifully illustrated by authors knowing the trade. A brief summary on the technique to implant cardioverter-defibrillators rounds up this section. These procedures will be around for a long time for sure.

After this, the attention is turned to a representative of balloon valvuloplasty. Let us not forget that interventional cardiology started with transcatheter valvuloplasty for stenoses. The mitral valve represents the most common target for percutaneous valvuloplasty these days, although the stock of patients in industrialized countries is limited. Rheumatic disease has been eradicated for decades and the reservoir of patients with secondary mitral stenosis is largely exploited. This is not (yet) the case for third world countries, where post-rheumatic mitral stenoses still abound.

Finally, a glimpse at the 'heart on the thigh' catches the eye. What has been predicted for more than 40 years but never considered really possible has become reality. The left ventricle can be not only supported but downright replaced for several weeks by a percutaneous intervention. You will have to read the chapter to come to believe it.

To live up to the name Atlas, the book is replenished with pictures. Authors and editors have gone to a great deal of trouble to select the best and reproduce them at the highest possible quality. Again, not unlike with the Sunday paper, you may decide to look at the pictures before lunch and pick it up again after lunch to read some or all of the text that comes with the pictures. You will have to try this concoction to be the judge of it. Your opinion may be mixed but you will have to admit that the book is different.

Bernhard Meier, MD
July 2004

# Abbreviations

2D  two dimensional

A  atrial sensing/pacing

(L/R)A  (left/right) atrium

(d/p)Abl  (distal/proximal) ablation catheter

(L/R)AC  (left/right) anterior cranial (view)

ACC  American College of Cardiology

ACT  activated clotting time

ADP  adenosine diphosphate

AF  atrial fibrillation

A. fem  femoral artery

ANF  atrial natriuretic factor

(L/R)AO  (left/right) anterior oblique (view)

AR  sensed atrial event within refractory period

AS  sensed atrial event

ASA  atrial septal aneurysm

ASD  atrial septal defect

ASH  asymmetric septal hypertrophy

AV  atrioventricular

bpm  beats per minute

Brugada-S  Brugada syndrome

BS  bystander site

CABG  coronary artery bypass grafting

CAD  coronary artery disease

CFI  collateral flow index

CI  central isthmus site

CK  creatine kinase

CPS  cardiopulmonary support

CS  coronary sinus

CT  computed tomography

CVP  central venous pressure

D  diastole

DCA  directional coronary atherectomy

DCM  dilated cardiomyopathy

DFA  deep femoral artery

DFT  defibrillation threshold

ECG  electrocardiogram

EGM  intracardiac electrocardiogram

ELCA  excimer laser coronary angioplasty

ESC  European Society of Cardiology

EV  Eustachian valve

f  fibrillation waves

FA  false aneurysm

FVT  fast ventricular tachycardia

GP  glycoprotein

HCM  hypertrophic cardiomyopathy

HF  heart failure

HNCM  hypertrophic nonobstructive cardiomyopathy

HOCM  hypertrophic obstructive cardiomyopathy

HR  heart rate

HRA  high right atrium

HV  shock delivery by implantable cardioverter-defibrillator

ICD  implantable cardioverter-defibrillator

IL  inner loop site

(L/R)IPV  (left/right) inferior pulmonary vein

IVC  inferior vena cava

IVUS  intravascular ultrasound

L   length

LAA   left atrial appendage

LAD   left anterior descending coronary artery

LCX   left circumflex coronary artery

LM   left main stem

LMWH   low molecular weight heparin

LO   location only

LQTS   long-QT syndrome

L-VAD   left ventricular assist device

LVEF   left ventricle ejection fraction

LVP   left ventricular pressure

MI   myocardial infarction

MR   magnetic resonance

NSVT   nonsustained ventricular tachycardia

Oa   anatomic orifice

Oe   echocardiographic orifice

Os   ostium

P   P-wave

PA   pulmonary artery

$P_{ao}$   mean aortic pressure

PCI   percutaneous coronary intervention

PET   positron emission tomography

PFO   patent foramen ovale

PI   proximal isthmus site

PLAATO   percutaneous left atrial appendage occluder

$P_{occl}$   mean distal coronary occlusive pressure

PTCA   percutaneous transluminal coronary angioplasty

(e)PTFE   (expanded) polytetrafluoroethylene

PTSMA   percutaneous transluminal septal myocardial ablation

PVP   pulmonary venous potential

R   ventricular sensing

RB   right bundle

Ref   reference catheter

RF   radiofrequency

RPM   revolutions per minute

RVC   right ventricular cardiomyopathy

Rx   therapy delivered by implantable cardioverter-defibrillator

S   systole

SAM   systolic anterior motion

Sat   oxygen saturation

SCD   sudden cardiac death

SFA   superficial femoral artery

SP   septum primum

(L/R)SPV   (left/right) superior pulmonary vein

SS   septum secundum

ST   sinus tachycardia

Stim   stimulation catheter

SVC   superior vena cava

SVT   supraventricular tachycardia

TA   tricuspid annulus

TEC   transluminal endarterectomy catheter

TOE   transoesophageal echocardiography

TS   tachycardia sensed event

UAP   unstable angina pectoris

US   ultrasound

V   ventricular sensing/pacing

(L/R)V   (left/right) ventricle

VF   ventricular fibrillation

$V_{occl}$   distal occlusive coronary flow velocity

$V_{\o\text{-}occl}$   coronary flow velocity during vessel patency

VP   paced ventricular event

VS   sensed ventricular event

VT   ventricular tachycardia

W   width

# Chapter 1

# Invasive Assessment of the Coronary Collateral Circulation

*Christian Seiler,* MD

## Introduction

The coronary collateral circulation has been recognized for a long time as an alternative source of blood supply to a myocardial area jeopardized by ischaemia[1]. Numerous investigations have shown a protective role of well versus poorly developed collateral arteries, showing smaller infarcts, less ventricular aneurysm formation, improved ventricular function, fewer future cardiovascular events, and improved survival[2, 3] (**1.1**). Precise characterization of collateral vessels has become increasingly important, since new therapeutic strategies for the promotion of collateral vessels, i.e. angiogenic and arteriogenic therapy, have been developed which await proper efficacy testing[4]. Ultimate coronary collateral assessment excluding confounding factors of forward flow requires an occlusion of the collateral receiving vessel, be it natural or artificial (**1.2**).

## Natural coronary occlusion model (chronic total occlusion model)

In the situation of a natural coronary artery occlusion without myocardial infarction, a well-developed collateral circulation must be the reason for the salvaged cardiac muscle (**1.3, 1.4**). The entire filling of a chronically occluded, collateral-receiving coronary artery from a collateral-supplying vessel (**1.3**) illustrates that the area at risk for infarction, i.e. a determinant of infarct size aside from vascular occlusion time, is closely and inversely dependent on collateral flow[5]. Thus, to detect normal ventricular wall motion (**1.4**) in the presence of a proximal or middle chronic occlusion represents a way of qualifying 'good' collateral flow.

## Artificial coronary occlusion model (angioplasty model)

At present, invasive cardiac examination is a prerequisite for reliable assessment of coronary collaterals. In the natural occlusion model, it is needed to confirm total vascular obstruction; in the artificial occlusion model, it is essential for briefly blocking the vessel using an angioplasty balloon catheter (**1.2**). Employing the angioplasty model, there are several qualitative and quantitative methods which can be used to characterize the collateral circulation[6].

### Angina pectoris and intracoronary electrocardiogram (ECG) during vessel occlusion

The simplest but rather imprecise way to qualify collateral vessels is to ask the patient about the presence of angina pectoris shortly before the end of arterial balloon occlusion. The predictive value of absent or present chest pain for collaterals sufficient or insufficient, respectively, to prevent ischaemia as detected by intracoronary electrocardiogram (ECG) is rather low. The use of an intracoronary ECG lead obtained via the angioplasty guidewire for collateral assessment provides a good representation of the pertinent myocardial area. Intracoronary ECG ST-segment changes of $>0.1$ mV constitute the definition of collaterals insufficient to prevent ischaemia in the respective myocardial territory (**1.5, 1.6**).

### Angiographic methods

The coronary angiographic method for collateral qualification most widely used is similar but not identical to the one first described by Rentrop and coworkers[7]. The latter provides a score from 0–3 for recruitable collateral vessels upon occlusion of the ipsilateral artery, the former an identical score for spontaneously visible collaterals without artificial vascular occlusion. The score describes epicardial coronary artery filling with radiographic contrast dye via collaterals as follows:

0: no filling;
1: small side branches filled;
2: major side branches of the main vessel filled;
3: main vessel entirely filled (**1.3**).

Clinically, the fact that only spontaneously visible collaterals are routinely scored further impairs the method's sensitivity, which is quite limited to begin with. Recruitable collateral vessel grading in the absence of chronic coronary occlusion, however, requires the insertion of two coronary catheters, i.e. one for balloon occlusion of the collateral-receiving vessel and one for injection of contrast dye into the collateral-supplying artery. An alternative, semiquantitative angiographic method consists of determining the number of heart beats during coronary occlusion needed to wash out the contrast medium; the contrast medium is retained in the vessel segment distal to the balloon because it was injected into the ipsilateral artery during balloon inflation. The contrast medium caught distal to the occlusive balloon can only be washed out by collateral flow (i.e. washout collaterometry[8]). A washout time of approximately 11 heart beats accurately predicts collaterals sufficient to prevent ischaemia during a brief coronary occlusion (**1.7, 1.8**).

### Intracoronary pressure or Doppler sensor measurements

Pressure or Doppler sensor tip angioplasty guidewires are available which are almost equivalent to regular guidewires in their handling properties. The theoretical basis for the use of intracoronary pressure or blood flow velocity measurements to determine collateral flow relates to the fact that perfusion pressure or velocity signals obtained distal to a balloon-occluded stenosis originate from collaterals (**1.5, 1.6, 1.9, 1.10**). The measurement of aortic and intracoronary pressure or velocity provides the basic variables for the calculation of a pressure-derived or velocity-derived collateral flow index (CFI), both of which express the amount of flow via collaterals to the vascular region of interest as a fraction of the flow via the normally patent vessel. Pressure-derived CFI is determined by simultaneous measurement of mean aortic ($P_{ao}$), mean distal coronary occlusive ($P_{occl}$), and central venous pressure (CVP) (**1.5, 1.6, 1.9**):

$$CFI = (P_{occl} - CVP)/(P_{ao} - CVP)$$

Velocity-derived CFI is measured by obtaining distal occlusive coronary flow velocity ($V_{occl}$) and coronary flow velocity during vessel patency ($V_{\emptyset\text{-occl}}$) taken at the same location and following occlusion-induced reactive hyperemia:

$$CFI = V_{occl}/V_{\emptyset\text{-occl}} \ (\textbf{1.10})$$

Pressure-derived and Doppler-derived intracoronary collateral measurements are regarded as the reference method for clinical assessment of coronary collateral flow.

**1.1** Cumulative rate of major adverse cardiac events in patients with stable coronary artery disease. During a follow-up period of almost 4 years, the event rate is significantly lower in patients with well versus those with poorly developed collateral vessels (where well developed collaterals are defined as invasively obtained CFI ‡25% of normal antegrade flow through the patent vessel, and poor collaterals are defined as CFI <25%). CFI: collateral flow index; MI: myocardial infarction; UAP: unstable angina pectoris.

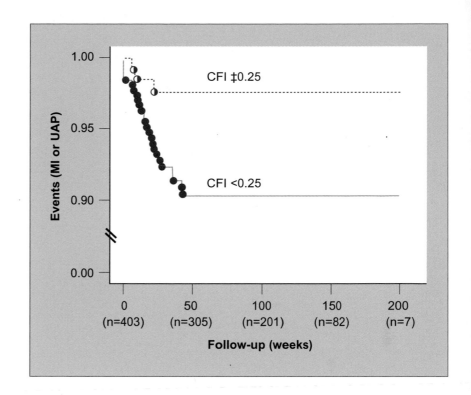

**1.2** Schematic drawing illustrating the condition under which the collateral supply to a specific coronary artery (i.e. the left circumflex coronary artery, LCX) can be assessed. Natural or artificial vascular occlusion of the collateral-receiving (i.e. ipsilateral artery, LCX) artery is mandatory for accurate assessment. LAD: left anterior descending coronary artery.

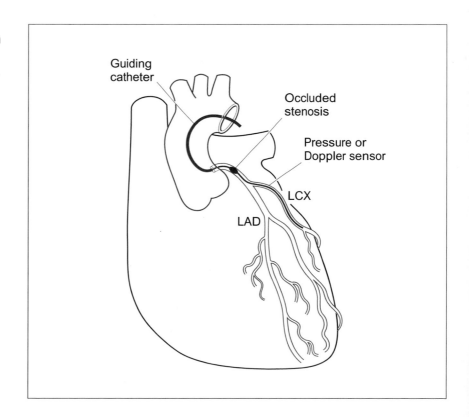

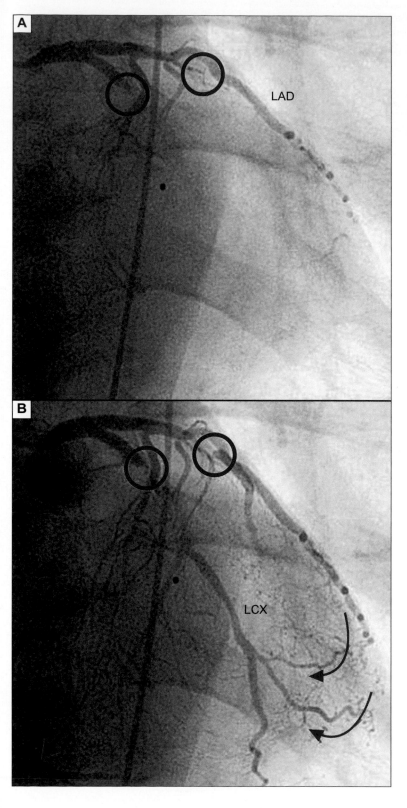

**1.3** RAO (right anterior oblique) (caudal view) coronary angiogram with injection of radiographic contrast medium into the left coronary artery. The two images are taken early (**A**) and late (**B**) during contrast injection. There are chronic total occlusions (red circles) of the proximal left circumflex (LCX) and the middle left anterior descending (LAD) coronary arteries, as well as retrograde filling via collateral vessels of the occluded right coronary artery (arrow). Complete retrograde filling with contrast (i.e. angiographic score 3; curved arrows) is documented for the LCX and LAD coronary arteries.

**1.4** Left ventricular angiogram of the patient in (**1.3**) obtained briefly after the coronary angiogram. RAO (right anterior oblique) view taken at end-diastole (**A**) and end-systole (**B**), illustrating an entirely normal systolic left ventricular function despite three-vessel coronary artery occlusion.

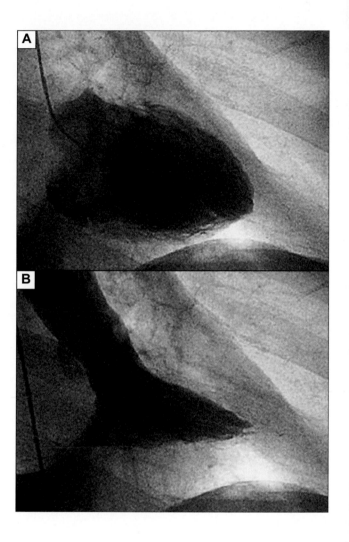

**1.5** Schematic drawing illustrating the principle of collateral assessment during coronary artery balloon occlusion using a sensor guidewire (blue line). This pressure or Doppler sensor is positioned distal to the occluded site. Pressure signals (except for venous back pressure) or flow velocity signals detected during vascular occlusion originate from collateral vessels supplying the blocked vascular region.

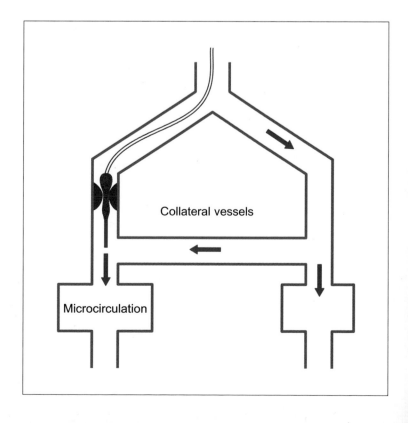

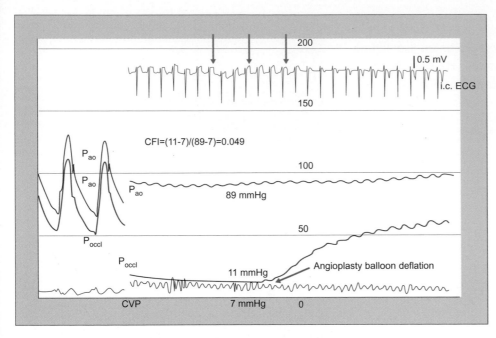

**1.6** Insufficient coronary collaterals: simultaneous recordings of an intracoronary electrocardiogram (i.c. ECG) lead (top), phasic (left side) and mean (right side) aortic ($P_{ao}$, mmHg), coronary occlusive ($P_{occl}$, mmHg), and central venous pressures (CVP, mmHg). $P_{ao}$ is gauged via the coronary guiding catheter, $P_{occl}$ via the pressure guidewire positioned distal to the stenosis to be dilated, and CVP via a right atrial catheter. To the right of the phasic pressure tracings obtained during coronary artery patency, mean pressures are recorded before, during, and after angioplasty balloon deflation. During balloon occlusion, there are marked ECG ST-segment elevations (arrows) indicating collateral vessels insufficient to prevent myocardial ischaemia. Collateral flow index (CFI) is calculated as follows: CFI = ($P_{occl}$ — CVP)/($P_{ao}$ — CVP).

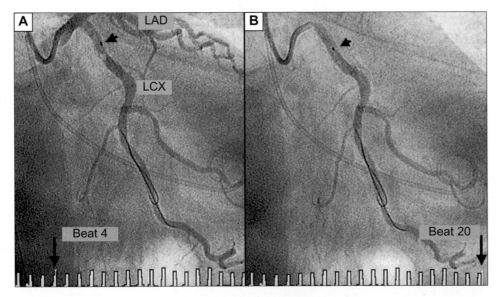

**1.7** RAO (right anterior oblique) coronary angiogram (projection: 27°, caudal 24°) showing slow contrast washout in the left circumflex (LCX) coronary artery. On the left (**A**), the situation 4 heart beats (large arrow) after angioplasty balloon inflation (position in the proximal LCX; black arrow head) is shown with the LCX distal to the balloon filled with radiographic contrast medium. On the right (**B**), the situation 20 heart beats (large arrow) after angioplasty balloon inflation is shown, whereby the radiographic contrast medium is not yet washed out distal to the balloon (arrow head). Collateral flow index in this case was 0.06. Contrast washout distal to the occluded vessel within 11 heart beats accurately separates collaterals sufficient from those insufficient to prevent ischaemia during brief coronary occlusion with 88% sensitivity and 81% specificity. LAD: left anterior descending coronary artery.

**1.8** RAO (right anterior oblique) coronary angiogram (projection: 17°, cranial 28°) showing fast contrast washout in the left anterior descending (LAD) coronary artery. On the left (**A**), the situation 4 heart beats (white arrow) after angioplasty balloon inflation (position in the mid-LAD; black arrow head) is shown, with the LAD distal to the balloon filled with radiographic contrast medium. On the right (**B**), the situation 10 heart beats (white arrow) after angioplasty balloon inflation (position in the mid-LAD; black arrow head) is shown, whereby the radiographic contrast medium is washed out distal to the balloon in the LAD but not in the diagonal branch. Collateral flow index in this case was 0.37. LCX: left circumflex coronary artery.

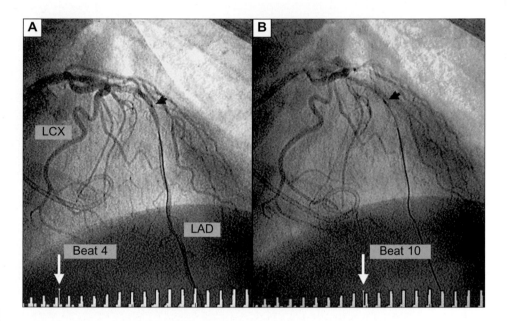

**1.9** Sufficient coronary collaterals: simultaneous recordings of an intracoronary electrocardiogram (i.c. ECG) lead (top), phasic (left side), mean (right side) aortic ($P_{ao}$, mmHg), coronary occlusive ($P_{occl}$, mmHg), and central venous pressures (CVP, mmHg). $P_{ao}$ is gauged via a 6 French coronary artery guiding catheter, $P_{occl}$ via a pressure guidewire positioned distal of a stenosis to be dilated, and CVP via a right atrial catheter. To the right of the phasic pressure tracings obtained during coronary artery patency, mean pressures are recorded during balloon inflation. During inflation, there are no ECG ST-segment elevations indicating collateral vessels sufficient to prevent myocardial ischaemia. Collateral flow index (CFI) is calculated as follows: $CFI = (P_{occl} - CVP)/(P_{ao} - CVP)$.

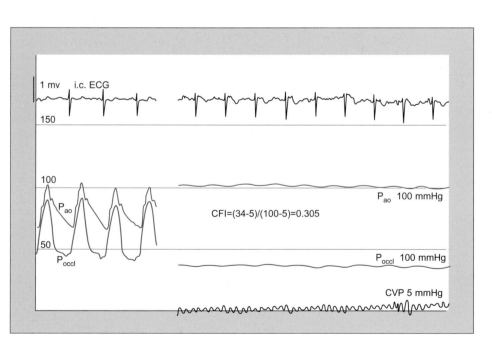

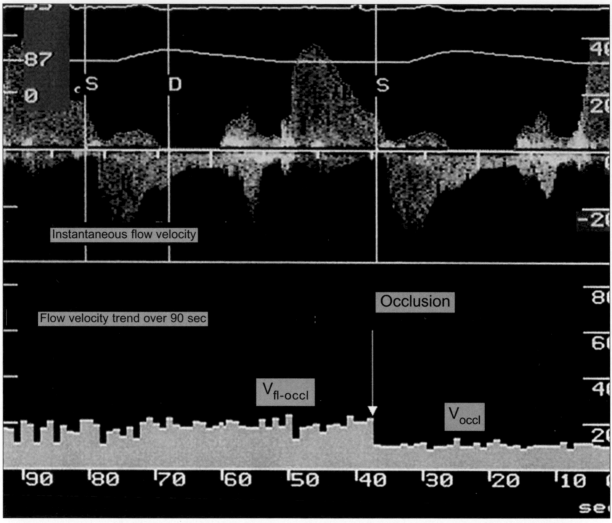

**1.10** Intracoronary Doppler flow velocity signals obtained distal to a balloon occluded vessel using a 0.014 inch, 20 MHz Doppler coronary guidewire. Upper panel: Instantaneous occlusive flow velocity profile recorded over time (horizontal axis). Bidirectional velocity signals indicate collateral flow towards and away from the Doppler sensor which is located at the tip of the guidewire. Lower panel: Flow velocity trend obtained over 90 seconds. Doppler-derived collateral flow index roughly corresponds to the ratio of flow velocity during occlusion ($V_{occl}$, cm/s) divided by flow velocity at the same site during vessel patency ($V_{fl-occl}$, cm/s).

## Conclusion

Well developed coronary collateral arteries in patients with coronary artery disease (CAD) mitigate myocardial infarcts with less ventricular aneurysm formation and improved ventricular function. They reduce future cardiovascular events, and improve survival. Myocardial infarct size is a product of coronary artery occlusion time, area at risk for infarction, and the inverse of collateral supply. Collateral arteries preventing myocardial ischaemia during brief vascular occlusion are present in one-third of patients with CAD.

Coronary collateral flow can be assessed only during natural or artificial vascular occlusion of the collateral-receiving artery. The entire filling of a chronically occluded, collateral-receiving coronary artery from a collateral-supplying vessel illustrates that the area at risk for infarction is closely and inversely dependent on collateral flow. The coronary angiographic method for collateral qualification describes epicardial coronary artery filling with radiographic contrast dye via collaterals, using a score from 0–3. An alternative, semiquantitative angiographic method consists of determining the number of heart beats during coronary occlusion needed to wash out the contrast medium caught in the vessel segment distal to the balloon due to pre-occlusion injection (washout collaterometry). Presently, the gold standard for clinical coronary collateral assessment is the measurement of intracoronary occlusive pressure-derived or velocity-derived CFI, which expresses collateral flow as a fraction of flow during vessel patency.

## References

1  Hansen JF (1989). Coronary collateral circulation: clinical significance and influence on survival in patients with coronary artery occlusion. *Am Heart J*, **117**:290–295.

2  Habib GB, Heibig J, Forman SA, Brown BG, Roberts R, Terrin ML, Bolli R (1991). Influence of coronary collateral vessels on myocardial infarct size in humans. Results of phase I thrombolysis in myocardial infarction (TIMI) trial. The TIMI Investigators. *Circulation*, **83**:739–746.

3  Billinger M, Kloos P, Eberli F, Windecker S, Meier B, Seiler C (2002). Physiologically assessed coronary collateral flow and adverse cardiac ischemic events: a follow-up study in 403 patients with coronary artery disease. *J Am Coll Cardiol*, **40**:1545–1550.

4  Seiler C, Pohl T, Wustmann K, Hutter D, Nicolet PA, Windecker S, Eberli FR, Meier B (2001). Promotion of collateral growth by granulocyte-macrophage colony-stimulating factor in patients with coronary artery disease: a randomized, double-blind, placebo-controlled study. *Circulation*, **104**:2012–2017.

5  Reimer KA, Ideker RE, Jennings RB (1981). Effect of coronary occlusion site on ischemic bed size and collateral blood flow in dogs. *Cardiovasc Res*, **15**:668–674.

6  Seiler C, Fleisch M, Garachemani A, Meier B (1998). Coronary collateral quantitation in patients with coronary artery disease using intravascular flow velocity or pressure measurements. *J Am Coll Cardiol*, **32**:1272–1279.

7  Rentrop KP, Cohen M, Blanke H, Phillips RA (1985). Changes in collateral channel filling immediately after controlled coronary artery occlusion by an angioplasty balloon in human subjects. *J Am Coll Cardiol*, **5**:587–592.

8  Seiler C, Billinger M, Fleisch M, Meier B (2001). Washout collaterometry: a new method of assessing collaterals using angiographic contrast clearance during coronary occlusion. *Heart*, **86**:540–546.

# Chapter 2

# Frugal Coronary Angioplasty

*Bernhard Meier,* MD

## Introduction

The most outstanding attribute of percutaneous transluminal coronary angioplasty (PTCA), today mostly referred to as percutaneous coronary intervention (PCI), is its frugality compared with coronary artery bypass surgery, an advantage which should not be given up lightly. This chapter in this practical compendium focuses, therefore, on how best to keep PCI frugal without losing efficacy or quality. A simple and straightforward approach in medical therapy is generally also cost-efficient. Cost has become a major issue in medical care in virtually all societies and it will remain one for good.

## Evolution of coronary angioplasty

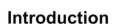

In 1964, Dotter and Judkins published a method to improve blood flow through narrowed peripheral arteries by forcefully passing the stenoses with catheters of increasingly large diameters[1]. As simple as the method was it implied that the size of the puncture hole be commensurate with the final lumen achieved. Andreas Roland Grüntzig, the father of coronary angioplasty, was not the only one to think of a balloon to render the method more practicable. Yet he was the only one who listened to a plastic expert first. Polyvinyl chloride was recommended as the working material[2]. The Grüntzig balloon dilatation catheter was successfully used in a few hundred peripheral arteries before Grüntzig managed to miniaturize it for use in the coronary arteries. In 1976, the coronary balloon was ready for a first attempt but it waited for over a year for a suitable patient. This may sound strange today. However, coronary angiography of yesteryear was restricted to patients resistant to a triple drug regimen against angina pectoris. Consequently, it almost exclusively yielded triple vessel disease with a damaged myocardium. The author was a fortunate witness of the first PCI procedure, which took place on September 16, 1977, at the University Hospital of Zurich, Switzerland. As the resident responsible for a 38-year-old male patient with recent onset of angina, the author presented Grüntzig with the coronary angiogram showing an isolated discrete stenosis of the left anterior descending coronary artery, with a conserved left ventricular function. Grüntzig promptly obtained oral informed consent from the patient who agreed readily to become the world's first PTCA patient. He was sharing the room with a patient recovering from coronary artery bypass surgery, the only therapeutic alternative.

What took place in the calm but somewhat tense atmosphere of the catheterization laboratory that day was a small step for Grüntzig but a huge step for mankind. Unlike the first landing on the moon 9 years earlier, this small step was going to have a definitive impact on mankind by changing medicine with the aid of a new prodigy, coronary angioplasty, the nidus and mainstay of interventional cardiology. Grüntzig died in a plane crash only 8 years later in 1985. His procedure was blessed to become the most important therapeutic intervention in medicine of industrialized countries. The first case was a full immediate success and the lesion was to be removed for the next 26 years (**2.1**), if not for good.

Coronary angioplasty admittedly had shortcomings, such as technical failures, acute complications like abrupt vessel closure, and recurrences within the initial months. However, these were more than compensated for by its virtues. The procedure is rapid and easy, turning a severely incapacitated patient into a fully functioning human being within a few hours and perhaps not even necessitating a night at the hospital. It results in virtual freedom from subsequent myocardial infarctions after a lesion has been successfully dilated. Late recurrence is practically inexistent, once the initial 6 months have not produced a stenosing scar at the dilated site. The procedure is easily repeatable in case of a necessity for the same or for further coronary problems, and there is a growing economic role of the industry built around the procedure (hospital facilities, production plants, medical education activities, publications). Millions of people benefit every year from this invention, be it as patients, as contributors, or both.

About 5 years after the introduction of this therapy modality, the respective activities had gained the necessary momentum around the world. At the same time attempts at improving the technique multiplied. They were welcome but they also rendered the procedure more intricate and jeopardized its frugality. None of them, shy of the coronary stent in its own frugality, was going to play a lasting role (**2.2**). Not even the stent markedly impacted on the leading role of the classical indication for coronary angioplasty, i.e. the treatment of a single coronary vessel. Single vessel angioplasty as propagated by Grüntzig from the start, accounted for over 80% of procedures at all times (**2.3**).

At least, the stent holds undisputable potential for making the procedure more safe. However, it failed to improve the complication figures in the European registry except for the decreasing need for emergency bypass surgery (**2.4**). The occlusive dissections bailed out by stent implantation should have reduced mortality and the occurrence of myocardial infarction. Yet stents are more prone to distal embolization phenomena, side branch occlusions, and late thrombotic occlusions. This forfeits their otherwise clear-cut advantage, in case they are overused. The trend to a reduced need for emergency bypass surgery had already started before the stent era and was based in great part on the recognition that emergency surgery improved the situation only in a few patients suffering a complication of coronary angioplasty. The severage from a mandatory surgical stand-by enhanced the frugality of coronary angioplasty and paved the way to use *ad hoc* angioplasty in the majority of cases (**2.5**).

To combine diagnostic coronary angiography and angioplasty makes perfect sense. While this option was initially frowned upon for ethical reasons and hampered by the poor resolution of X-ray equipment, necessitating processing and assessing 35 mm cine films for decision making, these caveats are no longer of essence. The cognizance of the general public, let alone patients with coronary artery disease, of the risks and benefits of coronary angioplasty is widespread and preliminary informed consent for an optional therapeutic add-on procedure can be obtained before the beginning of the diagnostic part of the catheterization. The resolution of modern digital coronary angiography laboratories is excellent and does no longer need to be improved by off-line processing.

The advantages of *ad hoc* angioplasty in terms of cost savings, sparing a second arterial puncture or even hospital stay, and reducing sick leave are obvious. At the author's centre *ad hoc* angioplasty is the rule. The only exceptions are cases referred from other centres. Institutions still adhering to performing diagnostic studies and angioplasty in separate sessions may have logistic reasons. In the Netherlands, only a minority of centres performing coronary angiography are approved for coronary angioplasty. Patients would refuse to have the diagnostic study done in a noninterventional centre, if the interventional centre offered a combined procedure. This would severely penalize the majority of cardiac centres and imbalance the respective medical coverage of the country. Some centres do not get adequate reimbursement to continue their activity if the procedures are combined. In other centres, there are purely diagnostic invasive cardiologists who have to refer their patients internally to therapeutic invasive cardiologists not necessarily available every day. The author strongly supports the concept of all invasive centres also performing therapeutic procedures, and of all invasive doctors also being trained in coronary angioplasty, unless they are working in a surrounding where an interventional colleague can be summoned to continue the case at all times.

**2.1** Site of first coronary angioplasty on September 16, 1977 before the procedure (inset) and at the latest follow-up angiogram on December 7, 2000 (23 years later).

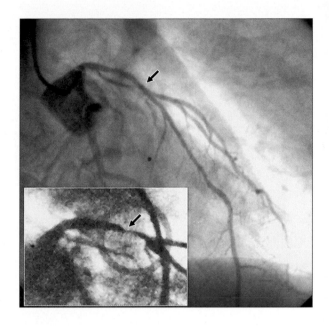

**2.2** Frequencies of PTCA (percutaneous transluminal coronary angioplasty) and associated procedures since its inception (modified from Bertrand and Serruys, personal communication).

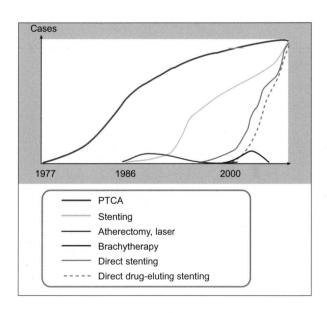

**2.3** Percentage of multivessel angioplasty performed in one session in a European registry, representing 27 countries with more than 570 million people and 530,000 coronary angioplasty procedures in the year 2000.

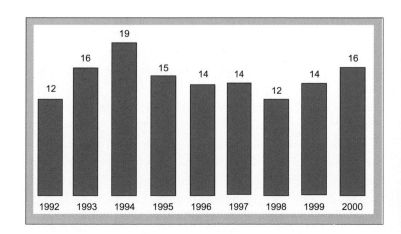

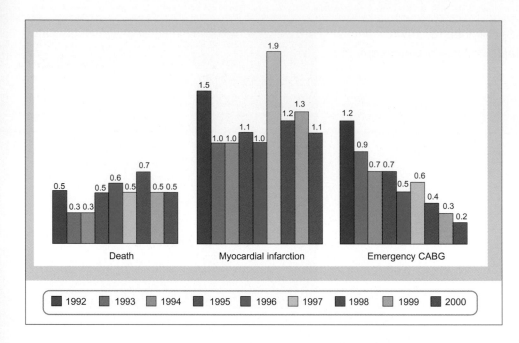

**2.4** Percentage of reported complications with coronary angioplasty in the European registry defined in (**2.3**). Emergency CABG (coronary artery bypass grafting) denotes the need for immediate coronary artery bypass grafting for a complication occurring during the procedure.

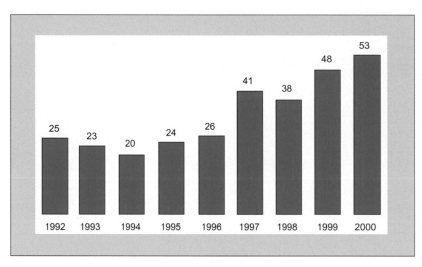

**2.5** Percentage of *ad hoc* angioplasty (angioplasty performed during the same session as the diagnostic coronary angiogram) in the European registry defined in (**2.3**).

## Tips and tricks to keep coronary angioplasty low cost

Besides the pivotal organizational policy to treat all cases *ad hoc* and to do them at the earliest normal working time period unless clinical facts impose an emergency intervention, several small technical details allow cost saving without sacrificing quality. *Table 2.1* offers an overview.

Should a need for emergency pacing arise, the arterial access can be used for either coronary pacing using the coronary guidewire (**2.6, 2.7**) or left ventricular pacing using the standard 0.035 inch guidewire or the coronary guidewire (**2.8**). If pacemaker dependability persists beyond the procedure which is exquisitely rare, a venous temporary pacemaker can be introduced under the protection of arterial pacing.

The cases depicted in **2.9** and **2.10** are practical examples of how to conduct coronary angioplasty efficiently and at low cost. A 64-year-old female was hospitalized for unstable angina. Coronary angiography demonstrated an isolated subtotal stenosis of the left anterior descending coronary artery, with normal left ventricular function (**2.9**). The 4 French introducer sheath used for the diagnostic coronary angiogram and ventriculography was replaced with a 5 French left Judkins coronary guiding catheter, inserted directly through the skin. Its outer diameter without an introducer is slightly smaller than the outer diameter of the 4 French introducer (about 5.5 French). This may occasionally lead to some oozing during the procedure (particularly in the presence of high blood pressure) but results in only a tiny hole (1.7 mm) to close. For this, manual compression for about 10 minutes almost always suffices, particularly if only 5,000 U of heparin are employed as is an acceptable routine for all cases of percutaneous coronary interventions. The lesion was dilated with a single 3.0 mm balloon inflation at 14 bar. Angiographic aspect (stent-like appearance) and flow were excellent and the patient was ambulated 3 hours later.

A 71-year-old male presented with unstable angina pectoris for 2 weeks, 22 years after single saphenous vein coronary artery bypass grafting to the left anterior descending coronary artery. Coronary angiography revealed a subtotal stenosis in the body of the bypass graft with the proximal native coronary artery occluded and a normal left ventricular function (2.10). The 4 French introducer sheath used for the diagnostic coronary angiogram and ventriculography was again replaced with a 5 French coronary guiding catheter (right Judkins), inserted directly through the skin. The lesion was dilated with a single 4.0 mm balloon inflation at 10 bar, yielding to 4 bar. The angiographic result 2 minutes after this inflation was pleasing, and the patient was ambulated 3 hours later.

Stenting of such short lesions in light of a good balloon result would carry an increased risk of distal embolization with poor distal run off but would not markedly reduce the risk of restenosis estimated at <20%. Moreover, it would introduce a hazard of subacute stent thrombosis. If the result had been unsatisfactory, a stent of up to 5.0 mm diameter could have been implanted through the 5 French catheter.

Even more complex cases can be handled in this thrifty but efficient fashion as shown in **2.11**. A 59-year-old male patient was admitted for worsening angina pectoris. He had had three previous coronary interventions 6–7 years earlier at another institution, where a stent had been placed in his proximal left anterior descending coronary artery. A follow-up angiogram at the same institution 5 years ago had diagnosed a take-off stenosis of the codominant left circumflex coronary artery, but an intervention was deemed too risky.

## Table 2.1 Tips to keep angioplasty frugal

*Personnel*
- 3 people needed, 2 at the table and 1 in the room.

*X-ray equipment*
- Biplane equipment, more expensive to buy but a real time saver.
- State-of-the-art digital imaging enhancement.
- Still frames to accelerate path finding.

*Table set-up*
- 2 spoke manifold (dye and pressure).
- No unnecessary instruments such as venous introducer for emergency pacing, blade holder, mosquito to spread incision.
- No intracoronary drugs (apply nitrates per spray).

*Technique*
- Small guiding catheters (avoid need for closure device).
- Reshape wire rather than replacing it.
- Use balloons in a logical sequence.
- Amplatz or multipurpose guiding catheters used if both coronary arteries have to be approached.
- Plan stenting carefully to avoid waste.
- Use dye frequently but in small amounts to find the way.
- Use expensive medications only when necessary.
- Do not measure activated clotting time (ACT).

*Aftercare*
- Mobilize as quickly as possible.
- Discharge as soon as possible.
- Keep vocational rehabilitation short.
- Emphasize secondary prevention to avoid medical cost in the future.

Coronary angiography was performed through a 4 French introducer sheath through the right femoral artery. Three significant lesions were diagnosed. One was at the take-off of the first diagonal branch (leaving from the stented segment), one was at the take-off of the left circumflex coronary artery (already diagnosed 5 years earlier but more severe now, partially produced by the proximal end of the stent in the left anterior descending coronary artery), and one was in the posterior descending branch of the right coronary artery. An intravenous bolus of 5,000 U of heparin was given. The patient had already received two sprays of nitroglycerine at the beginning of the diagnostic part of the procedure. The 4 French introducer was replaced by a 5 French left Amplatz 2 guiding catheter, again without using a sheath.

A 2.5 mm balloon catheter was introduced over a standard 0.014 inch coronary guidewire first into the take-off lesion of the first diagonal branch. The reason to start with this lesion was that the noninflated balloon was deemed to have the highest chance of passing through the stent. After an inflation at 10 bar the result was satisfactory. The same wire and the same balloon were used to dilate the take-off stenosis of the left circumflex coronary artery. This time the balloon was inflated at 20 bar to increase its outer diameter as this site was significantly larger. Again the result was satisfactory. The same guiding catheter was flipped over to the right coronary artery. The same balloon was introduced over the same guide wire into the posterior descending branch and successful balloon angioplasty was performed using an intermediate pressure (about 15 bar).

Although the risk of restenosis in one of the three sites could have been reduced by the use of stents, in particular drug-eluting stents, none of the lesions except for the one in the proximal left circumflex coronary artery is of great importance. Stenting this particular lesion would have involved the left main stem and distorted the entrance of the proximally located stent in the left anterior descending coronary artery. Therefore, the procedure would have become more complex and dangerous in order to reduce the risk of restenosis, which probably is only about 20% with the technique used.

While the case already affords considerable savings using but one guiding catheter, one balloon catheter, and one wire for angioplasty of three lesions in three vessels, even more material can be saved if a left Amplatz 5 French guiding catheter is introduced in the groin without an introducer from the start of the diagnostic procedure, as has been described[3].

Functional assessment of the collateralization status can be carried out in all these procedures without added cost. The technique of washout collaterometry is depicted in (**2.12**); this technique is applicable to all vessels and lesions, requires no additional material except for a small amount of contrast medium, and informs reliably about ipsi- and contralateral collaterals. The concept is further explained in Chapter 1.

**2.6** Coronary pacing during angioplasty. The negative pole of an ordinary temporary pacemaker unit is connected to the end of the coronary guidewire and the positive electrode is connected to a large surface electrode attached to the body of the patient. This may be a leg contact for the electrocardiogram (ECG, lower insert) or a separate skin patch. The coronary guidewire needs to be inserted deeply into a muscular branch of the respective coronary artery for good contact (upper insert). The output is first set at maximum and then reduced but kept above the pacing threshold. The outside connection can be accomplished manually, with an alligator clamp, or with a dedicated torquer-plug (centre circle).

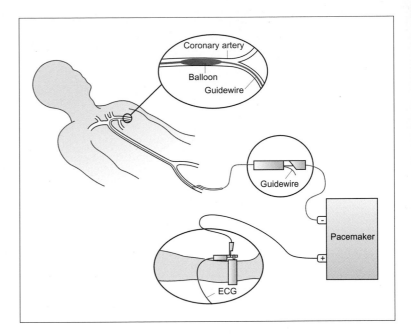

**2.7** Complete atrioventricular block with ventricular asystole during balloon occlusion of a right coronary artery. The blood pressure drops towards zero and the situation is remedied by coronary pacing re-establishing blood pressure promptly. Atrioventricular conduction resumed after balloon deflation.

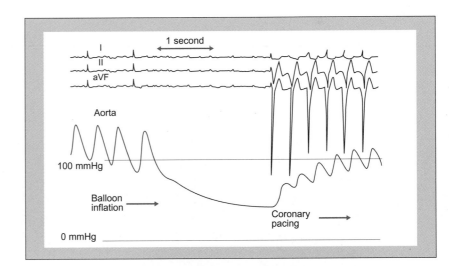

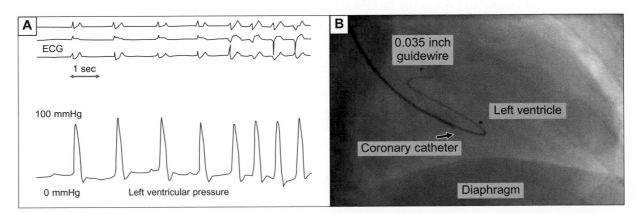

**2.8** Sinus arrest with slow ventricular rhythm (**A**) during diagnostic coronary angiography in a patient with severely impaired left ventricular function. Left ventricular pacing carried out via the standard 0.035 inch guidewire inserted through a coronary catheter into the left ventricle (**B**), immediately normalized the cardiac rhythm. ECG: electrocardiogram.

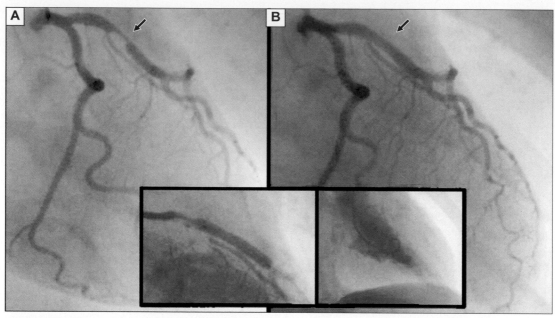

**2.9** RAO (right anterior oblique) view of a proximal stenosis (arrow) in the left anterior descending coronary artery before (**A**) and after (**B**) simple balloon angioplasty with a 3.0 mm balloon (left insert) inserted through a 5 French guiding catheter used without an introducer sheath. The right insert depicts the normal left ventricle at end-systole.

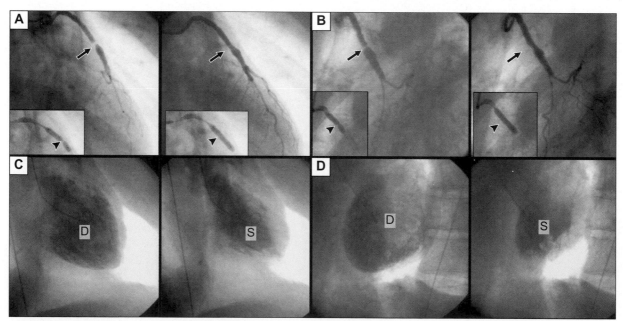

**2.10 A** RAO (right anterior oblique) view of a 22-year-old saphenous vein bypass graft to the proximally occluded left anterior descending coronary artery with a short but subtotal stenosis (left panel, full arrow). The 4.0 mm balloon inserted through a 5 French guiding catheter (without an introducer sheath) yielded to about 4 bar (inserts, arrow heads) and the result was good (right panel, full arrow). **B**: LAO (left anterior oblique) view of the process described in **A**. **C**: RAO view of the left ventricle in diastole (D) and systole (S), documenting a preserved function. **D**: LAO view of the left ventricle in diastole (D) and systole(S), again documenting a preserved function.

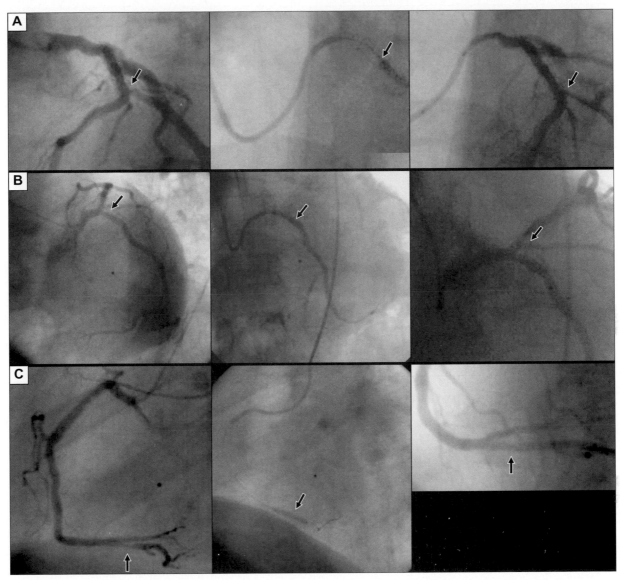

**2.11 (A)** LAO (left anterior oblique) view of the take-off stenosis of the first diagonal branch (arrow, left panel). Inflation of a 2.5 mm balloon at 10 bar is performed (arrow, centre panel) and the angiographic result shown (arrow, right panel). **(B)** Subtotal stenosis at the take-off of the left circumflex coronary artery (arrow, left panel). The same 2.5 mm balloon is inflated at 20 bar in this lesion (arrow, centre panel). A simultaneous dye injection during initial balloon inflation retains dye in the distal vessel. The fact that this dye has not washed out after 30 seconds proves the absence of collaterals from both the left and right coronary arteries. The right panel shows a good result after balloon angioplasty (arrow). **(C)** Stenosis of the posterior descending branch of the right coronary artery (arrow, left panel), dilated with the same 2.5 mm balloon at 15 bar (arrow, centre panel) with a good angiographic result (arrow, right panel).

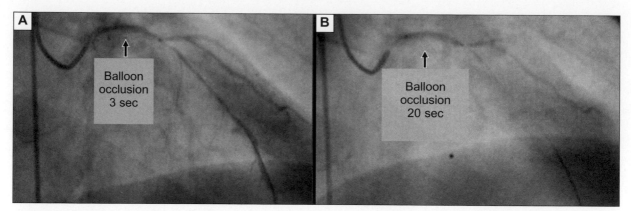

**2.12** Assessment of collateralization by washout collaterometry. The left panel (**A**) shows the situation of a left anterior descending coronary artery (LAD) 3 seconds after inflating a balloon proximally to block the artery (arrow), while simultaneously injecting contrast material. The contrast material caught distal to the balloon (which blocks antegrade flow once fully inflated) will inform about collateral inflow over the following seconds. The right panel (**B**) shows that at 20 seconds of balloon blockage, the LAD has been cleared of the contrast medium by collateral washout but not the large diagonal branch also blocked by the balloon. This proves collateralization of the former and no collateralization of the latter vessel. With this method ipsilateral and contralateral collaterals are accounted for. Ipsilateral collaterals could also be assessed by injecting contrast material into the left circumflex coronary artery while blocking the LAD, and looking for distal opacification of the latter. Direct demonstration of contralateral collaterals, however, would necessitate a simultaneous injection into the right coronary artery via a separately introduced right coronary catheter.

## Standard and optional equipment and procedures

*Table 2.2* lists what is standard and cannot be given up for simplification as it might negatively impact on the result of the procedure. Optional equipment is also listed. They add cost. They may be fancy, but can be deleterious to the result in some cases, or neutral in others. Some may be beneficial but only so exceptionally that they still can be foregone.

The covered stents may come in handy in case of a rupture of a coronary vessel. If a small vessel is concerned, the covered stent may be implanted in the main vessel at the take-off of the ruptured vessel. Finally, it can also remedy two annoying peripheral complications of coronary angioplasty, i.e. false aneurysms and arteriovenous fistulae at the femoral puncture site (**2.13**).

In particular, the low volume operator should stick to the standard instruments and techniques and stay away from optional methods. In a modern catheterization laboratory, a single or maybe two lines of guiding catheters, guidewires, and balloon catheters with and without stents, plus a limited

pharmacy including modern adenosine diphosphate (ADP) and glycoprotein (GP) IIb/IIIa antagonists suffice. The recommendation to use more expensive nonionic contrast medium may question the quest to curb cost. However, the negative effects of ionic contrast medium, such as negative inotropy and the tendency to produce bradycardia and nausea, are such nuisances that the higher price of noninonic contrast media is well invested.

The left ventricular assist system TandemHeart discussed in the final chapter is listed under standard equipment in *Table 2.2*. The brackets indicate that it is by no means a standard, yet. The TandemHeart is currently the only nonsurgical device that can replace left ventricular function completely, provided the right ventricle still functions. The device even maintains life during ventricular fibrillation, but right ventricular function has to be restored for long-term survival. The TandemHeart has realized a 40-year-old idea[4]. It harvests oxygenated blood from the left atrium and pumps it via a centrifugal pump on the thigh of the patient back into the lower aorta. In cases of severe or complete left ventricular failure, the aortic valve may remain closed and the entire body is perfused by the system which can achieve an output of 4 l/min at the maximum speed of about 7,000 revolutions per minute (RPM). The TandemHeart can be inserted, run, and removed percutaneously under local anaesthesia of the groin with a fully awake patient (see Chapter 9). To declare the TandemHeart a standard in frugal angioplasty may appear controversial. However, in contrast to other gadgets listed as optional, the TandemHeart is a potential life saver. It should at least be a standard for high volume angioplasty operators, even if they subscribe to a frugal angioplasty policy.

On the optional side, laser has failed to find any worthwhile niche in coronary angioplasty. Even the initially promising laser wire for chronic total occlusions is no match for dedicated conventional wires (stiff wires, ball-tip wires, hydrophilic wires) for this indication. Directional atherectomy has proved more complication prone, including a higher recurrence rate than plain balloon angioplasty. It is certainly no match for balloon angioplasty with stenting.

Rotational angioplasty (rotablator) solves an occasional case resistant to balloon inflation pressures at 30 bar when even the toughest balloons rupture. A centre without the technique may refer such cases (less than 1/100) to a larger centre. The cutting balloon is discussed in the paragraph of in-stent restenosis below. It has no place in the standard armamentarium. Thrombus extractors have such small indication niches that they are hardly worth mentioning.

Local drug delivery by catheter has proved too tedious, but has had a revival with drug-eluting stents. With them the drug is applied locally in a simple fashion. Intravascular ultrasound is advocated by many as a diagnostic tool with impact on the result. Scientific proof is lacking, the technique is costly and fairly intricate, and complications clearly overshadow any potential benefits. Hence, intravascular ultrasound is at best an option and can be ignored, unless scientific protocols call for it. The same holds true for physiological assessment of coronary flow or flow reserve with Doppler or pressure wires. Assessing the haemodynamic significance duplicates (more or less) the history taking or a stress test. If the patient reports angina and, particularly, if this is reproducible on a treadmill or a bicycle and accompanied by electrocardiogram (ECG) changes, the haemodynamic significance of the most conspicuous lesion(s) is sufficiently proved. Invasive assessment may confirm this but at extra cost and risk.

**Table 2.2 Standard and optional equipment and techniques for coronary angioplasty**

*Standard*
- State-of-the-art digital X-ray equipment.
- State-of-the-art coronary guiding catheters.
- State-of-the-art coronary guidewires.
- State-of-the-art balloon catheters.
- Stents:
  — Drug-eluting stents.
  — Covered stents.
- Nonionic contrast medium.
- (• Percutaneous left ventricular assist device.)

*Optional*
- Measurement of activated clotting time (ACT).
- Intracoronary nitrates.
- Laser debulker.
- Laser wire.
- Directional atherectomy.
- Rotablation.
- Cutting balloon.
- Thrombus smashers, absorbers.
- Local drug delivery catheters.
- Intravascular ultrasound.
- Doppler wire.
- Pressure wire.
- Methods to assess plaque vulnerability.
- Angioscopy.
- Brachytherapy.
- Puncture site closing devices.
- Intra-aortic balloon pump.
- Percutaneous cardiopulmonary support.
- Distal protection devices.

Moreover, relying on the haemodynamic significance of a coronary lesion is a misjudgement. Flow reduction by a lesion causes angina (which is a nuisance rather than a threat) but it only feebly predicts whether hard end points such as infarction or death are likely to be caused by this lesion later on, let alone at what point in time this may occur. To assess this prognostically important aspect of a coronary lesion much more sophisticated methods would have to be used (*Table 2.3*).

None of these methods has reached clinical routine application. None of them is likely ever to be added to the standard techniques in frugal angioplasty. The price paid for assessing a plaque may be higher than that for invasively treating it. Moreover, if the plaque proves unstable, the exact treatment will be done that would have been performed without assessing it. If, on the other hand, a plaque proves stable there is no guarantee that it will not turn unstable soon thereafter, perhaps even because of the invasive assessment.

Balloon angioplasty has been advocated to seal nonsignificant plaques, thereby removing or at last reducing their potential to subsequently cause a myocardial infarction. The principle of plaque sealing[5] is shown in (**2.14**). Plaque sealing of a nonsignificant stenosis is not yet an accepted procedure, but it is likely to become widespread with the availability of drug-eluting stents, in spite of a specific concern about this combination (see below). In contrast to an expensive assessment of the vulnerability of a specific plaque (*Table 2.3*), plaque sealing will avoid a disastrous case as shown in (**2.15**) swiftly, if performed during the diagnostic study. Plaque sealing may also save lifestyle type of events such as need for reintervention as depicted in (**2.16**).

The opposite concept of only dilating haemodynamically significant lesions has been investigated in a randomized trial[6]. At 2 years there was indeed no disadvantage of not dilating haemodynamically nonsignificant lesions. However, there was no advantage either. It can be assumed that the nondilated lesions simply are still awaiting their intervention, which could and probably should have been done during the initial angioplasty rather than being deferred. It is of note that the only death occurred in the group that was not dilated, from a plaque rupture of a nonsignificant lesion in a left anterior descending coronary artery a few months after randomization.

Angioscopy has been quite a useful tool but the industry is no longer offering the equipment as it was used too sparingly. The fact that the blood flow in coronary arteries not only needs to be blocked but the blood needs to be washed away to see is a great hindrance to the applicability of this method. Angioscopy survives in part at present in its subforms for assessment of plaque vulnerability (*Table 2.3*).

Brachytherapy has a proved effect in preventing restenosis. A rough calculation reveals, however, that 10 patients need to be treated in order to prevent one from having to come back for an additional angioplasty. Brachytherapy has no power to reduce prognostically relevant adverse events such as infarction or cardiac death. It merely acts on the nuisance of restenosis, which is more a lifestyle type of problem than life threatening. Only a few centres would have used this costly procedure for such a low yield. In the meantime, the advent of drug-eluting stents sent this therapy to oblivion. Brachytherapy would have had the same fate without drug-eluting stents, albeit more slowly.

Puncture site closure devices are not really necessary if procedures are performed with small guiding catheters. However, the convenience for the busy physician and physician assistant is indelible and the patient likes to ambulate earlier. Bleeding complications, have, however, not been reduced compared with manual or device compression.

## Table 2.3 Identification of vulnerable plaques

- Intravascular ultrasound.
  - —Three-dimensional reconstruction.
  - — Elastography (palpography).
  - — Intravascular ultrasound flow.
  - —Virtual histology.
- Angioscopy.
  - — Optical coherence tomography.
  - — Raman (near infrared) spectroscopy.
- Thermography.
- Positron emission tomography (PET).
- Computer tomography.
  - — Contrast.
  - — Ultrafast.
- Magnetic resonance (MR).
  - — Phase contrast.
  - — Nuclear.
  - — Intravascular.

The value of the intra-aortic balloon pump is highly overrated. It will never suffice when support is really needed. Where it seems to do good, support was probably not necessary in the first place. Percutaneous cardiopulmonary support, on the other hand, is a powerful assist system. Because of its intricacy it has not been accepted by the community of interventional cardiologists and is no longer available commercially. This fate is shared by the Hemopump system and may also happen to the currently advocated TandemHeart (see Chapter 9)

Distal protection devices are currently quite popular. The interest in these devices stems from carotid artery angioplasty. There distal embolization may result in catastrophic events such as aphasia, blindness, hemiplegia, or brain death. Although it is far from proved that these devices prevent more distal embolisms than they cause, doing something for distal protection is reassuring for the physician. In the coronary arteries, distal embolism may cause myocardial infarction or increase the loss of myocardium in ongoing infarction. An apparent sign of distal embolism is the so called 'no reflow phenomenon'. Again, no data clearly show the benefit of distal protection devices. To date their use, which is quite cumbersome and not without risk, is not uncommon particularly in angioplasty of old degenerated vein grafts. However, it is clearly acceptable not to use these devices at all and their final position in coronary angioplasty will depend on the outcome of randomized trials with different indications.

Figure **2.17** persiflages the current value of devices for coronary angioplasty. Among the ADP and GP IIb/IIIa antagonists, the thienopyridine copidogrel will probably dominate in the future. The ones up in the sun but with a doubtful outlook are distal protection devices as discussed above and the percutaneous left ventricular assist device, TandemHeart. Puncture site closure devices are a comfort item, not unlike the radial approach but they do not impact on the result and increase cost. They do not appear in the sunlight if frugality is first priority.

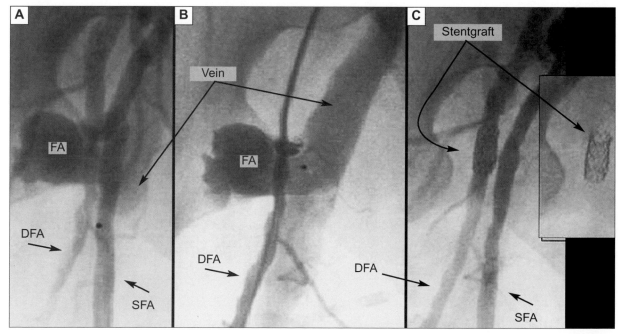

**2.13** False aneurysm and arteriovenous fistula in a 74-year-old male with six previous coronary angiograms through the right groin. (**A**) False aneurysm (FA) originating from the deep femoral artery (DFA). (**B**) It also communicates with the femoral vein (arteriovenous fistula). (**C**) After occlusion with a covered stent (stent graft, insert) from the contralateral side, both the deep and the superficial femoral arteries (SFA) are patent while the false aneurysm and the fistula have disappeared.

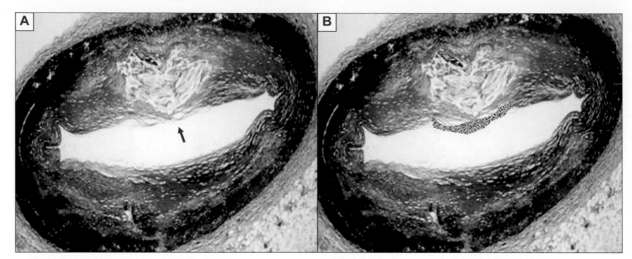

**2.14** Cross-section of a coronary artery with a nonsignificant narrowing of the lumen (no angina, no haemodynamic significance). The inherent risk of this plaque is a rupture at the thin fibrous cap (arrow, **A**). The right panel (**B**) shows the same site hypothetically after intentional rupture of this plaque with a balloon catheter and overgrowth of a new endothelial cap that is resistant to rupture and subsequent infarction (plaque sealing).

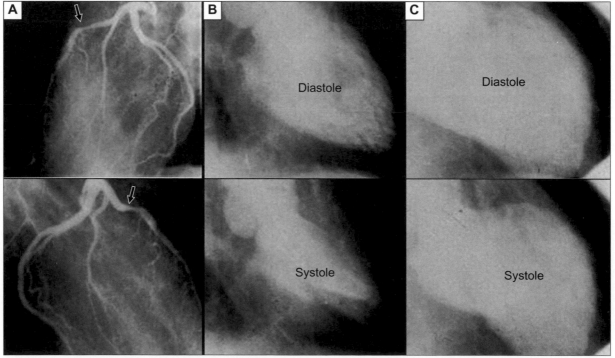

**2.15** Male patient (54 years) with atypical chest pain and a negative thallium stress test. The coronary angiogram shows a nonsignificant lesion in the proximal left anterior descending coronary artery (arrows, **A**) in a left (top) and right (bottom) anterior oblique projection. The ventricular function is normal (top: end-diastole; bottom: end-systole; **B**). Exactly 1 month later, the patient suffers an acute anterior myocardial infarction which he survives. However, his left ventricular function is completely ruined (top: end-diastole; bottom: end-systole; **C**) and the patient subsequently requires heart transplantation.

**2.16** Successful coronary balloon angioplasty (percutaneous transluminal coronary angioplasty, PTCA) of a tandem stenosis in the proximal left anterior descending coronary artery (upper left panel, pre-PTCA) with a good result (lower left panel, post-1st PTCA). A nonsignificant lesion distal to the second diagonal branch (white arrows) is not dilated (Not done), although it could have been dealt with utilizing the same material as the proximal lesions. Two years later the patient presents with unstable angina and anterior changes in the electrocardiogram. As expected, the initially dilated lesions proved to be in perfect shape (OK, centre panel) but the distal lesion had now progressed to a subtotal stenosis (white arrow, centre panel). The patient was lucky not to have suffered a myocardial infarction. This lesion was treated with a second balloon angioplasty with a good result (right panel, post-2nd PTCA) and long-term follow-up. Although no irreversible clinical event was prevented in this case, plaque sealing of the distal lesions at the initial angioplasty would have been cost-efficient and more comfortable for the patient, avoiding his second intervention.

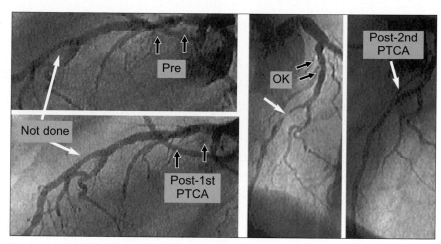

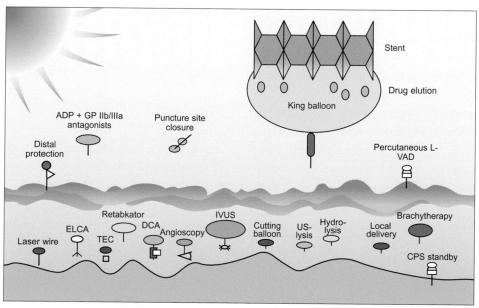

**2.17** Cartoon persiflaging the current value of different devices associated with coronary angioplasty. Many a device has been trying to break through the clouds to join the balloon catheter King Balloon crowned with the (now drug-eluting) stent in the bright sunlight. Some have had some time in the sunlight and have redescended. ADP: adenosine diphosphate; GP: glycoprotein; ELCA: excimer laser coronary angioplasty; TEC: transluminal endarterectomy catheter; DCA: directional coronary atherectomy; IVUS: intravascular ultrasound; US: ultrasound; L-VAD: left ventricular assist device; CPS: cardiopulmonary support.

## The role of stenting in frugal angioplasty

After an undeservedly slow start (**2.2**), stents have first emerged as the only worthwhile adjunct to balloon angioplasty in selected cases but have then gone on to indiscriminate overuse. Introduced as a bailout instrument to mend obstructive dissections after balloon angioplasty (occurring in about 5–10% of cases), they were found also to reduce restenosis. They eliminated the recoil or shrinking part of the restenosis process. This more than made up for the somewhat more active intimal proliferation after stent implantation. On the downside, they introduced subacute and late thrombosis at the treated site, something virtually unheard of with balloon angioplasty. They also brought about difficult-to-treat recurrences, the so-called in-stent restenoses (**2.18**). While a short in-stent restenosis poses no problem and is readily and lastingly treatable with balloon angioplasty, the diffuse type of in-stent restenosis is difficult to treat and yields a high re-restenosis rate.

For the melon seed phenomenon of the balloon slipping out of the in-stent lesion, the cutting balloon was recommended. It may be somewhat easier to keep in place during inflation, but this is no compensation for the significantly higher intricacy to get it to and into the lesion in the first place. The hope to reduce re-restenosis with the cutting balloon has been shattered by randomized trials. In-stent restenosis became basically the only indication for brachytherapy. However, for the reasons outlined above, it was hardly worth the trouble. The appearance of drug-eluting stents, reducing the risk of in-stent restenosis drastically, can be considered a real breakthrough. As for now, no disadvantages have been found to the two drug-eluting stents on the market (Cypher stent eluting sirolimus and Taxol stent eluting paclitaxel) compared with bare stents, except for their price.

Therefore, outside of rationed medical practice, every stent used should be a drug-eluting stent. Why should a patient be content to receive a stent with a higher restenosis risk if a better one is available that can be implanted without any extra effort? Figure **2.19** suggests, that the power of these stents to reduce restenosis has probably been conveyed in an exaggerated fashion. Nevertheless, it is there and placing a drug-eluting stent rather than a conventional stent requires neither additional time nor action during the procedure. The drug treatment afterwards may ask for prolonged use of clopidogrel, but that too is about to become commonplace.

In determining the advantages of using (drug-eluting) stents in frugal angioplasty, the following calculation should be taken into account. From the millions of plain balloon angioplasty procedures undertaken, 70% of lesions had a perfect result with a balloon alone. This means that they had no acute problem and never recurred. A stent cannot possibly improve on a perfect result but it may have a negative effect. Of the 30% balloon angioplasty procedures with either an acute problem or a restenosis, 5% would have had a problem in spite of a stent. This leaves 25% of lesions benefiting from implanting a stent. Of course, the problem lies in the unpredictability of a balloon angioplasty result, rendering it impossible to indentify these 25% in advance. An experienced operator assessing the result about 2 minutes after a balloon inflation will, however, be capable of narrowing down the lesions likely to benefit from stent implantation to about 50–60%.

An amateur or an evidence-based medicine buff not having completely digested the evidence will stent 100% of lesions. While the evidence is quite clear in terms of reducing the need for reintervention (remember, only a lifestyle type of problem) it shows overall no reduction of prognostically important events such as infarction or death, and may even increase these hazards in some subgroups[7]. While it makes perfect sense to stent immediately a conspicuous short but menacing dissection after balloon angioplasty, a long spiral dissection may be better left alone, as stenting will produce a good angiographic result only if the entire length of the vessel is covered (**2.20**). This harbours a considerable risk of subacute thrombosis or of hard-to-treat in-stent restenosis, probably even with modern antiplatelet agents and drug-eluting stents.

Other lesions not to stent are depicted in (**2.21**) and (**2.22**). A good indication for direct stenting, on the other hand, is shown in (**2.23**).

It should be kept in mind that in spite of two-pronged antiplatelet treatment, subacute and late stent thromboses occur in a few percent of cases, while balloon angioplasty is subject to the risk of vessel occlusion only for a few hours after the procedure. The implantation of a stent therefore trades in a beautiful aspect of the vessel and enhanced safety for the initial hours against a small but significant risk during the subsequent days and weeks. Then the patient is no longer in the hospital environment and therefore more at risk in the case of acute vessel closure than while still surveyed in the hospital close to the catheterization laboratory. Remember, drug-eluting stents do not improve that record as opposed to bare stents. Drug-eluting stents might at least on a theoretical basis be even be more prone to acute (polymer coating) or subacute thrombosis (coverage with new endothelium takes longer and is less complete). This concern has not materialized in the initial large scale randomized trials, but it is still lingering around and needs to be observed with the adoption of ubiquitous use of drug-eluting stents. There is a risk that subacute thromboses will increase by the fact that stenting will be used in a more cavalier manner (more and longer stents), assuming that restenosis is no longer an issue with drug-eluting stents. As a preventive measure, prolonged use of clopidogrel has been recommended and applied by most centres recently. Notwithstanding, drug-eluting stenting will increasingly be used, even in centres where it has not been used so far. Indications will be expanded towards mild lesions much in the sense of plaque sealing described above, albeit with probably the wrong technique.

It is unlikely that drug-eluting stents will considerably widen the indications towards the complex case for two reasons. First, it has to be reiterated that they do not improve safety of the procedure compared with conventional stents; second, not even introduction of conventional stents has had a significant impact on the percentage of multivessel angioplasty in a session (**2.3**). Therefore, a new upwards trend in the number of coronary angioplasty procedures predicted by many (**2.2**) will probably not take place. The additional mild cases treated may be compensated for by fewer reinterventions.

## Conclusion

Coronary angioplasty has got all it takes for an attractive medical therapy. It deals effectively with an extremely common illness. It turns nonsurgically active doctors into true healers with an immediate effect on the well-being of the patient, in many cases. It needs some dexterity and training but not too much. It offers technical challenges most often overcome thanks to excellent material and frequent opportunities to practice. It is well paid in many medical systems. There is a huge industry behind it eager to be kind to the direct consumers of their products, the angioplasty operators. Participation or even organization of pertinent meetings is generally enthusiastically welcomed by peers and sponsors. Although many publish in this field, numerous journals of the highest rank keep a vivid interest in this topic. Finally, coronary angioplasty calls upon the innovator in many an interventional cardiologist or even onlooker. Not a few of these innovations pay back at least for some time, although true break-throughs have been scarce since the crucial invention of the dilatation balloon by Grüntzig. In fact there has been only one, the introduction of the coronary stent in the mid-eighties and a partial one, its refinement to the drug-eluting stent, in the past few years.

One thing coronary angioplasty will never do, however often it is used, is replace coronary artery bypass grafting completely. Indications have not really changed much over the past quarter century. Indeed, Grüntzig's initial idea of how to use coronary angioplasty to its best has stood the test of time and is still valid. It is metaphorically depicted in (**2.24**).

As we will never detect and efficiently treat all coronary artery lesions as they come up, as some failures will always accompany PTCA (PCI), as many lesions may form simultaneously, and as the average age of the population keeps increasing, coronary artery bypass grafting will always have a place. Yet the majority of patients will move down the PTCA side of the plane (or bane) of life in **2.24** unless they are blessed with a life free of coronary artery disease altogether. PTCA being a repetitive thing even with the problem of restenosis tamed, it had better be swift and cheap, i.e. frugal.

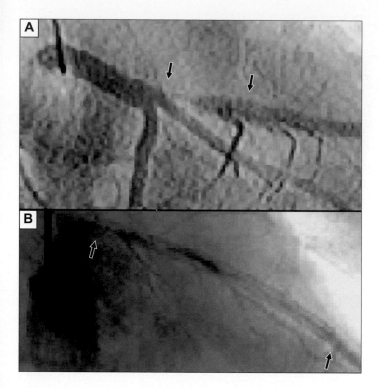

**2.18** Upper panel: Short in-stent restenosis 3 months after stent implantation. This lesion can easily be treated with simple balloon angioplasty. Lower panel: Diffuse in-stent restenosis 3 months after stent implantation. This lesion is extremely difficult to treat. The arrows denote the lengths of the stents.

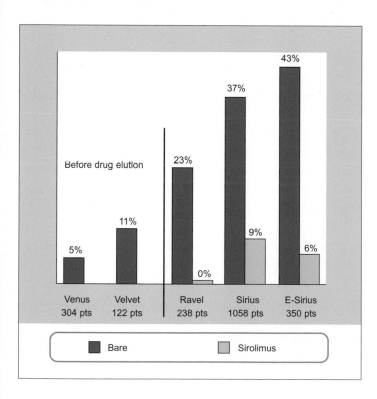

**2.19** Comparison of the reported restenosis rate of the Bx-Velocity stent before and after it was available in a drug-eluting version (Cypher stent). As observed often in medical research, a device (or compound) looks much better when it is compared with its predecessor than when it is compared with a new device (or compound) marketed to be its successor. There is really no explanation why the restenosis rate of the identical bare stents doubled or even tripled in core centre analyzed studies with comparable patients, once the drug-eluting version was available. The new version would have looked good even when compared with the restenosis rate of bare stents published before its availability, but the way it was finally presented made it more of a sensation.

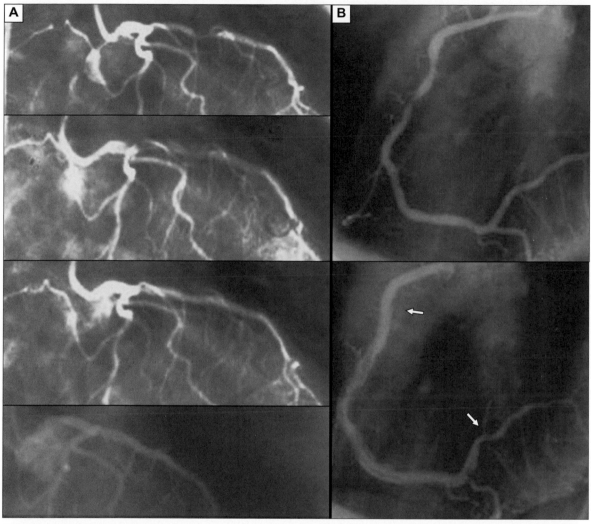

**2.20** Situations for stenting or not stenting. (**A**) After balloon angioplasty of a lesion in the mid-left anterior descending coronary artery (top) a conspicuous but circumscript dissection is visible (second from top). This is amended by stent implantation (third from top) and yields a good follow-up result (bottom). (**B**) A right coronary artery shows a long dissection after balloon angioplasty of a discrete lesion. The beginning and the end of the dissection are indicated by arrows (bottom right). Such a result can be left without stenting provided flow is unimpeded. If stenting is performed, it may be appealing but probably not wise to stent the entire length of dissection (full metal jacket). Stenting the entrance of the dissection only will in this case not be of much help either.

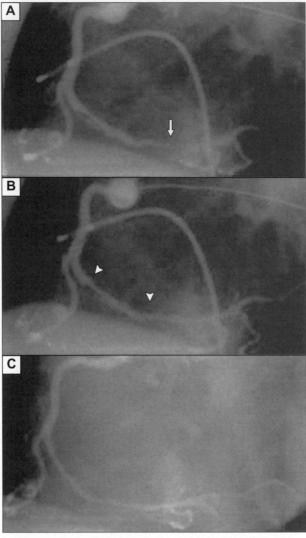

**2.21** Lesion not to stent. A subtotally stenosed right coronary is recanalized with balloon angioplasty of the culprit lesion (arrow, **A**). Flow is normalized but a long segment proximal to the stenosis looks stenosed because of accumulated thrombotic material (arrowheads, **B**). At follow-up angiography a few months later, the artery has completely cleared (**C**). The result with a long stent could only have been worse.

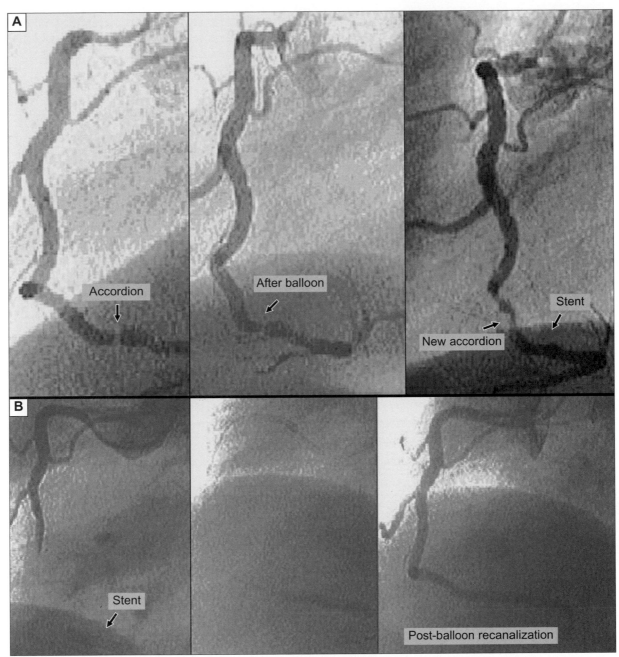

**2.22** (**A**) Lesion not to stent. A tortuous right coronary artery shows a kinking (accordion phenomenon, left panel). A balloon angioplasty does not change this finding (centre panel). After implantation of a stent the accordion has moved to the proximal end of the stent (right panel). (**B**) Ten days later the patient suffered an acute inferior myocardial infarction and the stent was found occluded (arrow, left panel). It was recanalized with balloon angioplasty (centre panel) with a good result (right panel) and long-term course. Accordion phenomena may also be induced by coronary guidewires or guiding catheters and should not be erroneously taken for lesions and stented.

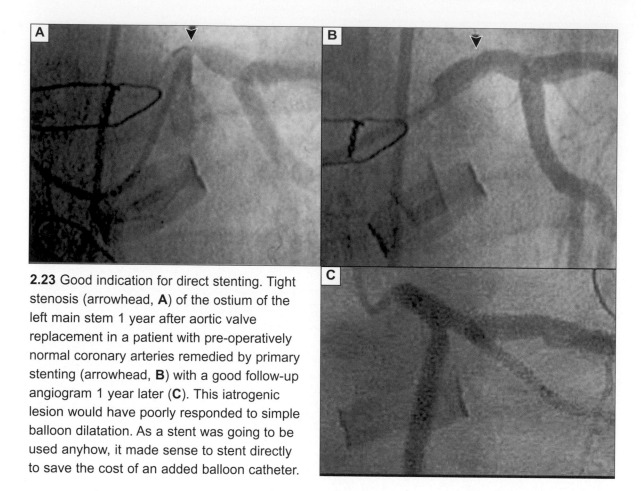

**2.23** Good indication for direct stenting. Tight stenosis (arrowhead, **A**) of the ostium of the left main stem 1 year after aortic valve replacement in a patient with pre-operatively normal coronary arteries remedied by primary stenting (arrowhead, **B**) with a good follow-up angiogram 1 year later (**C**). This iatrogenic lesion would have poorly responded to simple balloon dilatation. As a stent was going to be used anyhow, it made sense to stent directly to save the cost of an added balloon catheter.

# References

1 Dotter CT, Judkins MP (1964). Transluminal treatment of arteriosclerotic obstruction: description of a new technic and a preliminary report of its application. *Circulation*, 3:654–670.

2 Grüntzig A, Hopff H (1974). Perkutane rekanalisation chronischer arterieller verschlüsse mit einem neuen dilatationskatheter. *Dtsch Med Wochenschr*, 99:2502–2505.

3 Meier B (2004). Frugal coronary angioplasty, a case for the simple approach. *Catheter Cardiovasc Interv.*

4 Senning A, Dennis C, Hall DP, Moreno YR (1962). Left atrial cannulation without thoracotomy for total left heart bypass. *Acta Chir Scand*, 123:267.

5 Meier B, Ramamurthy S (1995). Plaque sealing by coronary angioplasty. *Catheter Cardiovasc Diagn*, 36:295–297.

6 Bech GJW, De Bruyne B, Pijls NHJ, *et al.* (2001). Fractional flow reserve to determine the appropriateness of angioplasty in moderate coronary stenosis: a randomized trial. *Circulation*, 103:2928–2934.

7 Brophy JM, Belisle P, Joseph L (2003). Evidence for use of coronary stents. A hierarchical bayesian meta-analysis. *Ann Intern Med*, 138:777–786.

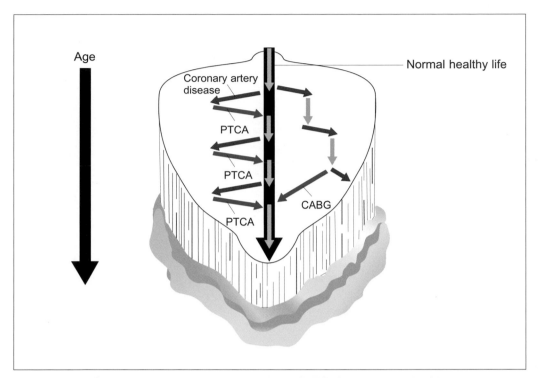

**2.24** Model of how to use coronary angioplasty (PTCA) best to deal with coronary artery disease during a lifetime. It can be called the c(o)urse of life. At birth, we are cast on a high plane on which to move invariably forward. Some day we will inevitably fall off the cliff. It is in everybody s interest to stay on or near the centre line, as any deviation from it carries the risk of a premature demise. Coronary artery disease, as any disease, can be characterized with this model. It may hit quite early in life with a first lesion (upper left red arrow). With a successful PTCA we will rejoin our healthy fellow age-mates on or near the centre line. Years or decades later, a second lesion may occur and the same form of therapy may again bring us back to the centre line, and so forth. Finally, we may achieve a normal life span thanks to PTCA which, however, has to be performed serially just as Gr ntzig had planned and predicted.

If the first manifestation of coronary artery disease is not invasively treated (upper right red arrow) a stable phase may follow nonetheless, thanks to modern drug treatment. However, life goes on closer to the dangerous precipice. With a second lesion, the same may take place but this time the proximity to the cliff becomes truly menacing. A third lesion may be fatal unless it is recognized early enough and treated with coronary artery bypass grafting (CABG), PTCA rarely being an option in these situations.

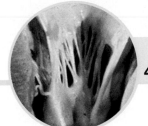

# Alcohol Ablation of Septal Hypertrophy

*Otto Hess*, MD, *Francesca Como*, MD, *and Thomas Wolber*, MD

## Introduction

Septal hypertrophy associated with outflow tract obstruction has been described in patients with hypertrophic cardiomyopathy; secondary forms have also been observed in elderly patients with long-standing hypertension[1]. Alcohol ablation has been used to reduce septal wall thickness at the site of outflow tract obstruction. The first successful alcohol ablation was performed by Sigwart in 1995 in a patient with hypertrophic, obstructive cardiomyopathy[2]. Hypertrophic cardiomyopathy (HCM) is a primary myocardial disorder with an autosomal pattern of inheritance, characterized by inappropriate myocardial hypertrophy[3, 4]. The prevalence of HCM in the general population has been estimated as 1:500, higher than was previously thought[4].

Several molecular genetic studies have described HMC as an heterogeneous disease of the sarcomere that involves more than 150 different mutations in at least 10 different contractile proteins[5, 6]. This genetic complexity leads to a wide diversity in cardiac morphology, pathophysiologic features, and clinical manifestations even in a single family cohort with clear implications for the prognosis[4, 6]. Annual mortality for HCM in unselected population has been reported at about 1%[7] and sudden death represents the most common cause. Sudden death is assumed to be due to ventricular arrhythmias but haemodynamic factors and myocardial ischaemia may also be involved.

The most common pattern of hypertrophy is asymmetric septal hypertrophy (**3.1**), whereas other localization, i.e. apical, mid-ventricular, or concentric hypertrophy appear to be far less frequent[6]. From a haemodynamic standpoint, HCM is classified into *obstructive* (HOCM) and *non-obstructive* (HNCM) forms. A third form, *apical hypertrophic cardiomyopathy* has been described which is relatively uncommon in Europe and USA, but is typically found in Japan. The dynamic obstruction can be extremely variable and may be present at rest or after provocation with amylnitrite or Valsalva manoeuvre. Thus, the complex hypertrophic process leads to a hyperdynamic left ventricle, typically small and irregularly shaped with enhanced systolic ventricular function, whereas diastolic function is impaired with increased filling pressures and delayed relaxation and abnormal filling rates. Myocardial stiffness is most commonly elevated. The major determinant of diastolic dysfunction in HCM is the degree and severity of left ventricle (LV) hypertrophy.

## Diagnosis

The most important tool to diagnose HCM is two-dimensional (2D) Doppler echocardiography This technique allows detection of three characteristic findings in HCM:

- Asymmetric septal hypertrophy (septal/posterior wall thickness ratio ≥1.5) = ASH.
- Dynamic LV obstruction with systolic outflow tract gradient.
- Systolic anterior motion (SAM) of the anterior mitral leaflet with concomitant mitral regurgitation.

The electrocardiogram (ECG) may be helpful for diagnosis because giant negative T-waves in the precordial leads have been described as typical for HCM, specifically for the apical form. Almost all patients with HCM show electrocardiographic signs of LV hypertrophy. Holter monitor testing may help to identify patients at risk for nonsustained or sustained ventricular tachyarrhythmias.

## Differential diagnosis

Asymmetric septal hypertophy may be seen in patients with long-standing arterial hypertension. Elderly, female patients with hypertension have been diagnosed with hypertensive hypertrophic cardiomyopathy. Diagnosis may be difficult and symptomatology is often similar to HCM, but elevated blood pressure may be diagnostic[1].

### Key points

- Always consider hypertrophic cardiomyopathy in young people and young athletes with signs of inappropriate LV hypertrophy or a history of syncope.
- Always rule out HCM in young patients with negative T-waves in the precordial leads of the ECG. Recommend 2D-Doppler echocardiography. Consider that coronary artery disease with negative T-waves (nontransmural infarction or hibernating myocardium) is rare in this age group.
- Myocardial fibre disarray and cellular disorganization are common in HCM and are not confined to the hypertrophied portions of the left ventricle, but may also be seen in regions with normal wall thickness.

## Therapy

Management of patients with HCM is directed toward alleviation of symptoms, prevention of complications (e.g. atrial fibrillation [AF]), and reduction in sudden cardiac death[7].

### Medical treatment

Management of HCM is directly dependent on the symptomatology of the patient and the presence or absence of outflow tract obstruction (**3.2**). Asymptomatic patients are usually not treated, except those with severe LV hypertrophy. Symptomatic patients should receive either calcium antagonists or beta-blockers. Both classes of drugs have been associated with symptomatic improvement, but

**3.1** Autopsy specimen of a patient with severe hypertrophic cardiomyopathy. The interventricular septum is massively hypertrophied (approximately 4 cm thickness) and the outflow tract severely narrowed (approximately 3—4 mm), with a thickened endocardium in the region of the mitral valve—septal contact.

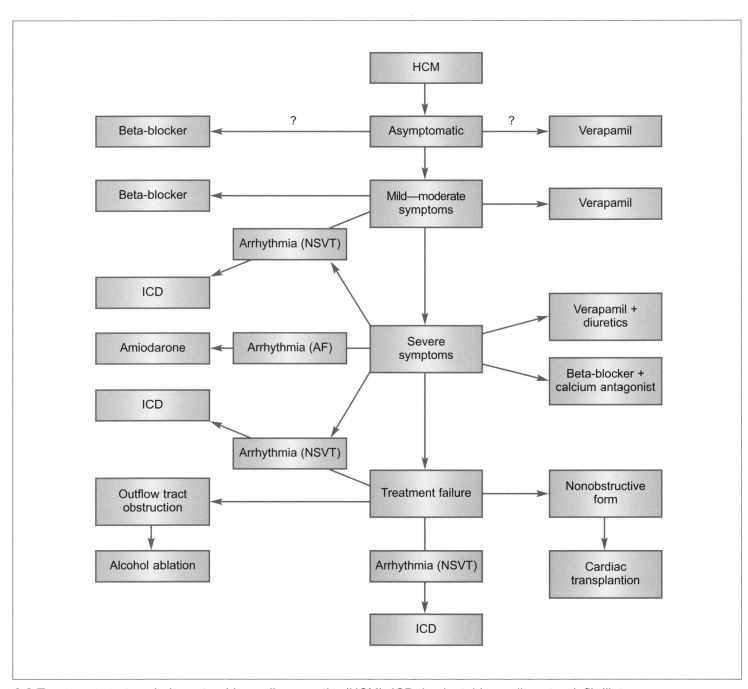

**3.2** Treatment strategy in hypertrophic cardiomyopathy (HCM). ICD: implantable cardioverter-defibrillator; NSVT: nonsustained ventricular tachycardia; AF: atrial fibrillation. (Courtesy of Hess[9].)

controlled studies which have documented a prognostic benefit are lacking. Diuretics have been previously thought to be contraindicated, but are currently used for patients with pulmonary congestion in combination with or without calcium antagonists or beta-blockers. HCM patients may be sensitive to rapid volume changes with a drop in cardiac output. Digitalis should generally be avoided unless AF or systolic dysfunction develops.

Therapy-refractory patients with severe outflow tract obstruction should be managed by interventional strategies such as alcohol ablation of the septum or surgical myectomy. Long-term follow-up after surgical myectomy has shown excellent results[8], but ventricular remodelling with dilatation of the left ventricle may become a problem in 15–20% of all patients. Patients with severe LV hypertrophy, recurrent syncopes, sustained and nonsustained ventricular tachyarrhythmias, a history of familial sudden cardiac death, and a genetic phenotype for an increased risk of premature death should be treated with an implantable cardioverter–defibrillator. Amiodarone may be used in patients with supraventricular (AF) and ventricular tachyarrhythmias, although in severe cases implantation of a defibrillator may be mandatory. Dual-chamber pacing has been used to reduce outflow tract obstruction, but plays a minor role today and may be limited for special indications such as complete atrioventricular (AV) block after alcohol ablation.

Treatment is indicated when the patient becomes symptomatic or LV hypertrophy is severe (**3.2**). Refractoriness to medical therapy usually indicates progression of the disease. At this point, the use of more aggressive therapies, such as alcohol ablation of the septum or surgical septal myectomy are indicated. Dual-chamber pacing for symptomatic relief and reduction of outflow tract obstruction has been used previously, but is not recommended at present for general use. However, insertion of implantable cardioverter–defibrillators is strongly advised in high-risk patients with a family history of sudden cardiac death, severe LV hypertrophy with nonsustained or sustained ventricular tachyarrhythmias, or syncopes.

## Complications

Strenuous exercise or competitive sports should be avoided in patients with HCM because of the risk of sudden death. Typically, sudden death occurs during or just after strenuous physical exercise. Atrial fibrillation as a cause of diastolic dysfunction with increased filling pressure and dilatation of the atria should be pharmacologically or electrically converted because of the haemodynamic consequences of the loss of atrial contraction on cardiac output. If sinus rhythm cannot be attained, oral anticoagulation is mandatory unless contraindications exist. Infective endocarditis may occur in about 5% of HCM patients and antibiotic prophylaxis is indicated. Infection typically occurs on the aortic or mitral valve or on the septal contact site of the anterior mitral leaflet.

### Alcohol ablation of the hypertrophic septum

Recently, alcohol ablation of the interventricular septum has been recommended as the treatment of choice to reduce or eliminate LV outflow tract obstruction. Outflow tract gradients of 30–50 mmHg at rest and 75–100 mmHg after provocation (extrasystole, isoproterenol infusion, or amylnitrite inhalation) qualify for septal ablation (**3.3**).

Two arterial catheters are introduced from the right femoral artery, a 4 French pigtail catheter for LV-angiography and continuous pressure (gradient) recording, and a 6 French guiding catheter for coronary angiography and alcohol ablation. A 6 French pacing catheter is introduced through the right femoral vein into the right ventricle for temporary pacing when needed. After installation of the catheters, coronary angiography is performed to identify the first or second septal branch (**3.4**) for alcohol ablation. A guidewire is then placed in either one of these branches and an over-the-wire balloon (1.5–2.0 mm diameter, 10 mm long) is advanced into the septal branch (**3.4B**). Then the balloon is inflated with 3–4 bar and echo contrast medium (1–3 ml) is injected (**3.5**) for identification of the target area (cave: papillary muscle, distal septum). Pure ethanol (1–3 ml) is then injected over 3–5 minutes to ablate the septum. Alcohol injection should be made slowly, and ECG changes (cave: AV-block III) watched carefully (**3.6**). Typically, the patient experiences chest pain, which may be mild or sometimes severe. All patients are pre-treated with 5–10 mg morphine and/or 1–2 mg midazolam when necessary. Many patients show immediate reduction or elimination of the pressure gradient (**3.3**) and the septum becomes akinetic in the 2D-echocardiogram. Approximately one-third to one-half of all patients show only minor reduction in pressure gradient, but higher doses of alcohol are not recommended because of the increased risk of developing AV-block III. In cases with no reduction in pressure gradient and only minimal haemodynamic changes, a second branch may be ablated. At the end of the procedure, all catheters are removed; however, the pacing catheter should be kept in place until the next morning or for approximately 12 hours following the intervention. At the authors' centre patients are monitored for at least 36–48 hours to watch for arrhythmias and late AV-block. Creatine kinase (CK) rise is usually between 500 and 1000 U/l but may rise to 1500 U/l in single cases. Hospital stay is around 2–3 days, but may be longer if pacemaker implantation is necessary.

### Ventricular remodelling

Follow-up examinations are recommended after 3 and 6 months with 2D-echocardiography (**3.7**) to measure pressure gradient and LV-remodelling (a decrease in wall thickness and reduction in LV muscle mass). The remodelling process may last up to 6 months before a definitive decision on the success of alcohol ablation may be taken or the indication for another intervention may be discussed.

Holter monitoring may be indicated in those with arrhythmias or suspected intermittent AV-block. Medical therapy with beta-blockers or calcium antagonists is required in most patients but may be discontinued later on, depending on clinical success of the intervention.

### Surgical treatment

Until 4–5 years ago septal myectomy had been considered as the treatment of choice for therapy-refractory patients with hypertrophic, obstructive cardiomyopathy[8, 9]. The introduction of alcohol ablation has changed this concept completely, and surgical resection of the septum is reserved for selected cases with combined procedures such as coronary bypass grafting or mitral valve repair.

## Prognosis and outcome

The clinical course in HCM is variable in many patients and may remain stable over many years. However, HCM patients with several risk factors such as a familial history of premature death, recurrent syncopes, severe septal hypertrophy (septal thickness >30 mm), or a genetic phenotype with an increased risk of premature death may show a poor outcome. Annual mortality rates have been reported to range between 2–3%, but may be higher in children[4, 6]. Clinical deterioration is often slow but clinical symptoms are poorly related to the severity of outflow tract obstruction. Generally, symptoms increase with age. The occurrence of AF is usually an indicator for diastolic dysfunction with increased filling pressures and dilated atria. Timely conversion of AF is often indicated because patients may become rapidly symptomatic.

## Conclusion

Percutaneous transluminal septal myocardial ablation (PTSMA) is a safe and effective procedure to achieve sustained reductions of intraventricular pressure gradients and LV septal thickness in HOCM. Late LV remodelling is associated with a further decrease in outflow obstruction and left atrial diameter with sustained benefits in clinical symptoms. Complications are rare but include the risk of development of transient (20–30%) or permanent (3–5%) AV-block.

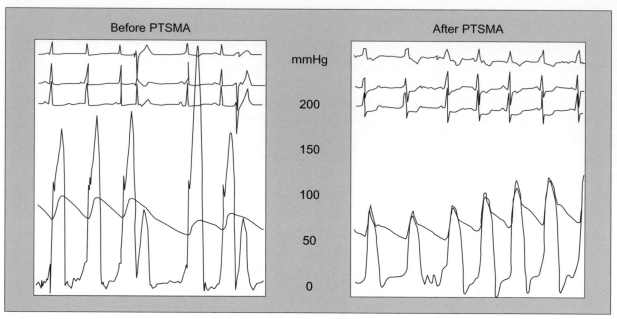

**3.3** Pressure recording in a patient with hypertrophic cardiomyopathy before and after alcohol ablation of the septum (PTSMA). Before the intervention there is a large pressure gradient at rest (75 mmHg ) and after post-extrasystolic potentiation (150 mmHg). The systolic pressure gradient disappears completely after alcohol ablation.

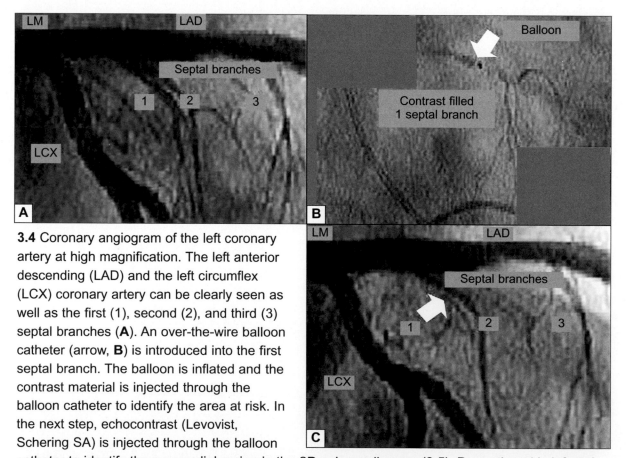

**3.4** Coronary angiogram of the left coronary artery at high magnification. The left anterior descending (LAD) and the left circumflex (LCX) coronary artery can be clearly seen as well as the first (1), second (2), and third (3) septal branches (**A**). An over-the-wire balloon catheter (arrow, **B**) is introduced into the first septal branch. The balloon is inflated and the contrast material is injected through the balloon catheter to identify the area at risk. In the next step, echocontrast (Levovist, Schering SA) is injected through the balloon catheter to identify the myocardial region in the 2D-echocardiogram (**3.5**). Pure ethanol is infused over 3—5 minutes which leads to reduction or elimination of outflow tract obstruction (**3.3**). The last angiogram (**C**) shows that the first septal branch has disappeared after alcohol injection (arrow). LM: left main stem.

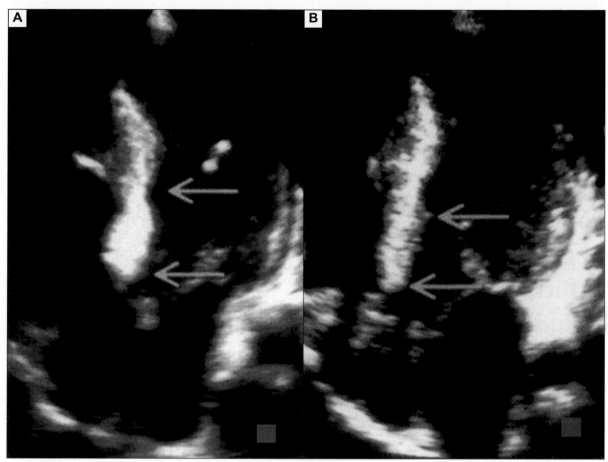

**3.5** 2D-echocardiogram before and after alcohol ablation. Arrows indicate septal hypertrophy after injection of echocontrast medium (**A**). Normalization of septal thickness 1 month after the intervention is shown (arrows, **B**). (Courtesy of Seggewiss and Faber[11].)

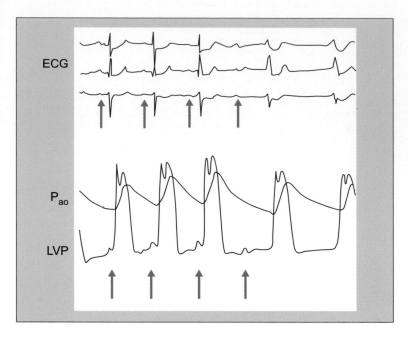

**3.6** Simultaneous electrocardiogram (ECG) and pressure recordings in a patient during alcohol ablation. Arrows indicate atrial contraction in the ECG (upper row) and left ventricular pressure curve (lower row). Occurrence of third degree atrioventricular (AV) block can be seen after the fourth atrial beat, with a left ventricular escape rhythm (bundle branch block). Three to four minutes after the occurrence of third degree AV-block a normal sinus rhythm was restored. $P_{ao}$: aortic pressure; LVP: left ventricular pressure.

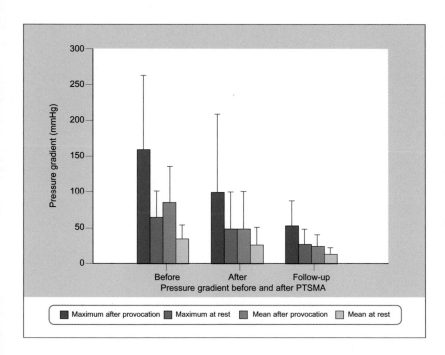

**3.7** Doppler echocardiographic pressure gradients before and after alcohol ablation (PTSMA) and during follow-up. Given are the maximal pressure gradients after provocation with amylnitrite (first bar), and at rest (second bar), mean pressure gradient after provocation (third bar) and at rest (fourth bar). Early after the intervention there is a significant decrease in pressure gradients by one-half, followed by a further reduction during follow-up (6 months) to one-third of the initial values. These data indicate that left ventricle-remodelling may take 3—6 months after successful alcohol ablation.

# References

1  Topol EJ, Traill TA, Fortuin NJ (1985). Hypertensive hypertrophic cardiomyopathy of the elderly. *N Engl J Med*, **312**:277–283.

2  Sigwart U (1995). Nonsurgical myocardial reduction for hypertrophic obstructive cardiomyopathy. *Lancet*, **346**:211–214.

3  Frank S, Braunwald E (1968). Idiopathic hypertrophic subaortic stenosis. Clinical analysis of 126 patients with emphasis on the natural history. *Circulation*, **37**:759–788.

4  Maron BJ, Gardin JM, Flack JM, *et al.* (1995). Prevalence of hypertrophic cardiomyopathy in a general population of young adults. Echocardiographic analysis of 4111 subjects in the CARDIA Study: Coronary Artery Risk Development in (Young) Adults. *Circulation*, **92**:785–789.

5  Maron BJ, Shen WK, Link MS, *et al.* (2000). Efficacy of implantable cardioverter–defibrillators for the prevention of sudden death in patients with hypertrophic cardiomyopathy. *N Engl J Med*, **342**:365–373.

6  Spirito P, Bellone P, Harris KM, *et al.* (2000). Magnitude of left ventricular hypertrophy and risk of sudden death in hypertrophic cardiomyopathy. *N Engl J Med*, **342**:1778–1785.

7  Wigle ED, Rakowski H, Kimball BP, Williams WC (1995). Hypertrophic cardiomyopathy: clinical spectrum and treatment. *Circulation*, **92**: 1680–1692.

8  Seiler C, Hess OM, Schoenbeck M, *et al.* (1991). Long-term follow-up of medical versus surgical therapy for hypertrophic cardiomyopathy: a retrospective study. *J Am Coll Cardiol*, **17**:634–642.

9  Schönbeck MH, Brunner-LaRocca PH, Vogt PR, *et al.* (1998). Long-term follow-up in hypertrophic obstructive cardiomyopathy after septal myectomy. *Ann Thorac Surg*, **65**:1207–1214.

10  Hess OM (2003). Risk stratification in hypertrophic cardiomyopathy. Fact or fiction? *J Am Coll Cardiol*, **42**:880–881.

11  Seggewiss H, Faber L (2000). Perkutane transluminale septale Myokardablation bei hypertropher obstruktiver Kardiomyopathie. In: Hess OM, Simon R, *Herzkatheter-Einsatz in Diagnostik und Therapie*, Springer Verlag, pp. 502–516.

# Chapter 4

# Percutaneous Closure of Patent Foramen Ovale

*Markus Schwerzmann, MD, Stephan Windecker, MD, and Bernhard Meier, MD*

## Introduction

The atrial septum is formed by two overlapping embryological structures: the left-sided fibrous septum primum, and the right-sided muscular septum secundum (**4.1**). During intrauterine life, the septum primum serves as a one-way valve and allows passage of blood from the umbilical vein entering through the vena cava inferior directly into the left atrium, bypassing the pulmonary circulation (**4.2**). The postnatal increase in left atrial pressure pushes the thin left-sided septum primum against the septum secundum, and closes the foramen ovale. Anatomic sealing follows in the ensuing months. In one-quarter of the population sealing is incomplete, giving rise to a patent foramen ovale (PFO) in adult life[1].

Excess atrial tissue may allow increased movement of the septum secundum depending on situational left and right atrial pressure. When the excursion is >15 mm in total, or >10 mm beyond the plane of the interatrial septum, an atrial septal aneurysm (ASA) is diagnosed (**4.3**, **4.4**). Echocardiography studies show an ASA in 2–4% of the population, frequently (50–70%) associated with a PFO[2] (**4.5**).

## Diagnosis

A PFO cannot be diagnosed by clinical examination. Multiplane transoesophageal echocardiography (TOE) with contrast injection is the investigation of choice for the diagnosis of a PFO. During the TOE, aerated colloid solution is injected into an antecubital vein, followed by flushing with 10 ml saline. Patients have to be coached to perform a Valsalva manoeuvre just before the injection with release after arrival of contrast in the right atrium, thereby increasing right atrial pressure with opening of a potential PFO. A good Valsalva manoeuvre is followed by bulging of the septum secundum into the left atrium. During Valsalva, both atria are poorly filled. After Valsalva, the right atrium is filled several seconds before the left atrium by the blood rushing into the thorax from the abdomen. The injection has to be repeated at least twice in two orthogonal echo-cardiographic planes. The diagnosis of a PFO requires crossing of bubbles from the right into the left atrium within four cardiac cycles after full opacification of the right atrium (**4.6**). Ideally, the bubble transit through the PFO is visualized directly. A prominent Eustachian valve (**4.7**) may collimate the blood flow through the vena cava inferior to the fossa ovalis (**4.8**), and may hamper correct diagnosis of a PFO by inhibiting opacification of this region after antecubital (i.e. via vena cava superior) contrast application (**4.9**). In this case, injection of contrast medium into a leg vein increases the diagnostic accuracy (**4.10**).

Transthoracic echocardiography with contrast injection has a sensitivity 50–80% of that with TOE[3, 4]. Transcranial Doppler sonography with antecubital contrast application is used by neurologists for detection of a right-to-left shunt. Right-to-left shunted microbubbles cause hyperintense audible signals during transcranial insonation of the middle cerebral artery. Localization of the shunt is not possible, and overall diagnostic accuracy is inferior to that with TOE[3]. The diagnostic yield of transcutaneous oxymetry (rapid and transient drop in saturation after release of a Valsava manoeuvre) (**4.11**) is under investigation.

If percutaneous PFO closure is planned, prior TOE is mandatory for exclusion of concomitant atrial septal defects and other potential sources of cardiac emboli.

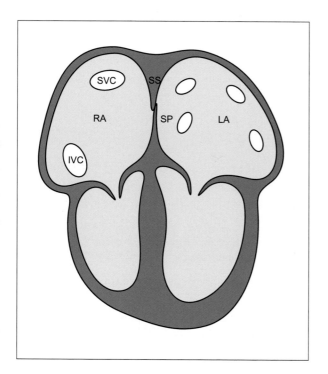

**4.1** After birth, left atrial pressure exceeds right atrial pressure and closes the foramen ovale. The circles in the left atrium indicate pulmonary veins. IVC: inferior vena cava; SP: septum primum; SS: septum secundum; SVC: superior vena cava; RA: right atrium; LA: left atrium.

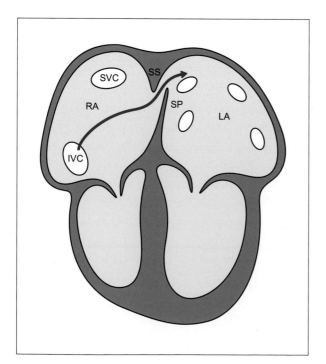

**4.2** If anatomical sealing is incomplete in adult life, situationally increased right atrial pressure opens the foramen ovale, i.e. a patent foramen ovale is present. Predominantly blood from the inferior vena cava will be shunted into the left atrium (red arrow). IVC: inferior vena cava; SP: septum primum; SS: septum secundum; SVC: superior vena cava; RA: right atrium; LA: left atrium.

**4.3** Increased mobility (double-headed arrow) of the septum primum due to an atrial septal aneurysm is frequently associated with a large patent foramen ovale. IVC: inferior vena cava; SP: septum primum; SS: septum secundum; SVC: superior vena cava; RA: right atrium; LA: left atrium.

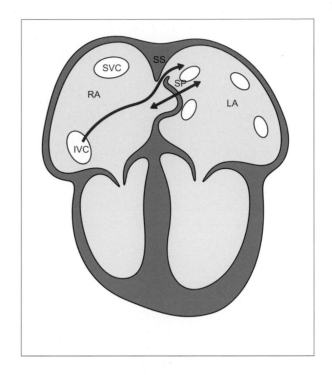

**4.4** Transoesophageal contrast echocardiography showing a foramen ovale closed at the moment but associated with an atrial septal aneurysm. LA: left atrium; RA: right atrium; SP: septum primum; 1: extent of the atrial septal aneurysm; 2: maximal protrusion of the atrial septal aneurysm in the right atrium beyond the imaginary plane of the atrial septum.

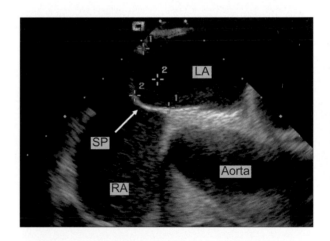

**4.5** Opening of the foramen ovale. ASA: atrial septal aneurysm: LA: left atrium; RA: right atrium; PFO: patent foramen ovale; SS: septum secundum.

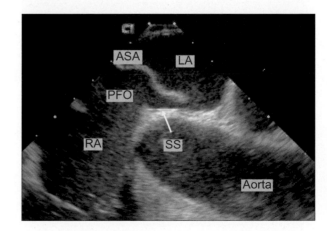

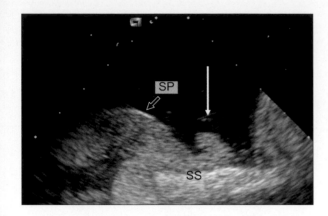

**4.6** Passage of aerated saline appearing as a cloud of bubbles through a large patent foramen ovale (arrow) in the presence of an atrial septal aneurysm. The patency of the foramen ovale can be semiquantitatively assessed by counting the number of bubbles in the left atrium on a still frame: small shunt (0—5 bubbles), moderate shunt (6—20 bubbles), large shunt (>20 bubbles). SP: septum primum; SS: septum secundum.

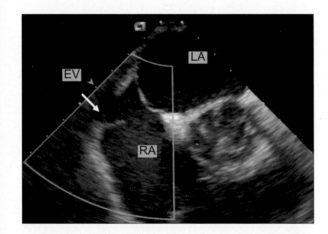

**4.7** A prominent Eustachian valve directs the inflow of the vena cava inferior (arrowhead) to the region of the fossa ovalis. EV: Eustachian valve; LA: left atrium; RA: right atrium.

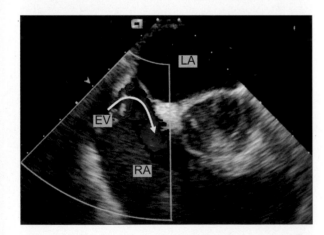

**4.8** Using Doppler sonography the deviation of the blood to the fossa ovalis by the Eustachian valve (EV) (blue colour) and its deflection (red colour) by the atrial septum can be demonstrated (arrow). LA: left atrium; RA: right atrium.

**4.9** After contrast injection into an antecubital vein, a negative contrast phenomenon is observed (arrow). It consists of superior vena cava flow being pushed off by the inferior vena cava flow. LA: left atrium; RA: right atrium.

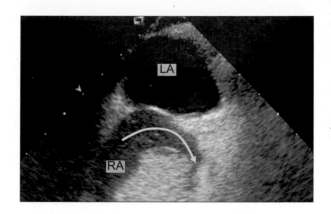

**4.10** Application of contrast medium via inferior vena cava to direct the bubbles to the region of fossa ovalis. This increases the sensitivity of the method.

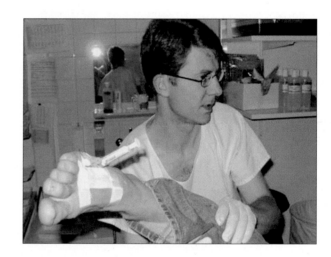

**4.11** Transcutaneous pulse oxymetry in a diver without any structural cardiac abnormalities but a patent foramen ovale (grade II). After release of the Valsalva manoeuvre (red arrow) a transient dip in transcutaneously measured oxygen saturation is repeatedly observed. HR: heart rate; Sat: oxygen saturation.

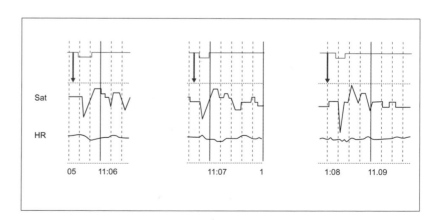

## Clinical relevance of a PFO

It has been estimated that about 750,000 strokes occur yearly in the USA. Stroke is the third leading cause of death after heart disease and cancer. About 80% of strokes are of ischaemic origin; of these, about one-third are cryptogenic. PFO has been associated with cryptogenic stroke. Pooled data in adults <55 years reveal presence of a PFO in 46% of such patients with cryptogenic stroke as compared with only 11% in matched controls[5–7]. Larger PFO size[8], and the presence of an ASA increase the risk of stroke[6]. Patients with cryptogenic stroke related to PFO are at risk for recurrence despite medical treatment, a risk again particularly pronounced in patients with a PFO and associated ASA[2]. Paradoxical embolism mediated by an intermittent right-to-left shunt has been suggested as the most likely stroke mechanism in this patient population[2] (**4.12, 4.13**). Current knowledge suggests that percutaneous PFO closure protects against recurrent strokes as well as medical antithrombotic treatment with acetylsalicylic acid or oral anticoagulation[9–11]. Randomized trials on the protective effect of percutaneous PFO closure in recurrent stroke patients are underway. Percutaneous PFO closure may be especially efficient in situations at higher risk of paradoxical embolism such as the presence of an ASA, an Eustachian valve directed toward the fossa ovalis, or a large PFO size[12].

Patent foramen ovale has also been related to orthostatic desaturation in the setting of the platypnoea-orthodeoxia syndrome[13], refractory hypoxemia in patients with right ventricular infarction[14], adverse outcome in patients with major pulmonary embolism[15], and decompression illness and ischaemic brain lesions in divers[16].

About 3–5% of the general population suffer from migraine with aura[17]. Recently, a higher prevalence of right-to-left shunt was observed in patients with migraine with aura compared to healthy controls[18, 19]. In addition, observational studies have shown a higher prevalence of migraine with aura in stroke patients with a PFO compared with those without[20, 21]. Patients with interatrial septal defects referred for percutaneous closure have incidentally found to report abolishment or marked improvement of migraine after intervention[22]. Currently, a study is ongoing to assess the effect of percutaneous PFO closure on frequency and impact of headache attacks in patients with migraine with aura.

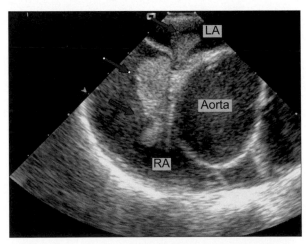

**4.12** Although paradoxical embolism through a patent foramen ovale (PFO) is a presumptive diagnosis most of the time, occasionally passage of a thrombus can be documented. In a 45-year-old male suffering from pulmonary embolism caused by a fragment breaking off the tail of the thrombus while it was lodged in the PFO, a 30 cm long thrombus (red arrow) was found at echocardiography. LA: Left atrium; RA: right atrium.

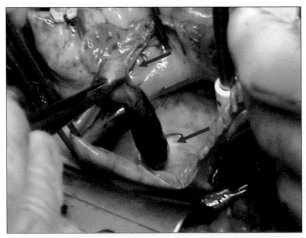

**4.13** The thrombus depicted in (**4.12**) (arrows) during surgical removal.

# Practice of percutaneous PFO closure

Patients are brought to the catheterization laboratory in the fasting state. The procedure is performed under local anaesthesia. Venous access is gained via the right femoral vein and the PFO is passed under fluoroscopic guidance, e.g. using a Multipurpose catheter. Using a standard or exchange wire, the Multipurpose catheter is exchanged for a 8–12 French trans-septal sheath according to the device selected. The Starflex device (NMT), the Amplatzer PFO Occluder (AGA), and the PFO Star device (EV3) (**4.14**) are most commonly used for PFO closure in the USA and Europe. After placing the trans-septal sheath in the left atrium, the left-sided device disk is unfolded and pulled back against the septum, thereby pulling the septum primum against the septum secundum and closing the foramen. The right-sided disk is then deployed and the device released. Prior to release of the device, its position is controlled using right atrial contrast angiography to delineate the atrial septum (**4.15–4.21**). Transoesophageal or intracardiac echocardiography guidance is used instead of, or in addition to, contrast injections at some centres (**4.22**). The correct position of the device can be assessed under fluoroscopy by looking for a straddling of the two device disks by the thick muscular septum secundum (**4.23**). This structure must be caught in between the device disks, thereby creating a so-called Pac-Man sign (**4.24, 4.25**).

All the different devices currently in use are available in several sizes; for instance the Amplatzer PFO Occluder is available as 18 mm, 25 mm, or 35 mm size. These sizes refer to the right atrial disk (**4.14**). Atrial septal anatomy and PFO size dictate device size. In the presence of an atrial septal aneurysm with very mobile septum primum and a large shunt, a device has to be chosen which covers all of the tunnel exit area (**4.26, 4.27**) and is safely straddling the septum secundum (**4.28**). This allows for a stable device position and complete sealing of the defect after device endothelialization. However, a large device often goes beyond, with additional rubbing of the device against the ascending aorta (**4.29, 4.30**). It may also lead to an unfavourable device profile in the right atrium, hampering device endothelialization, and may partially protrude into the superior vena cava inflow tract (**4.31, 4.32**). Therefore, the best policy is to use the smallest device providing a stable position and fully covering the defect (**4.33, 4.34**).

Meticulous handling is necessary to avoid air in the delivery system. Besides paradoxical air embolism, haematoma at the entry site, pericardial effusion after atrial perforation, embolization of the device in the pulmonary artery or left ventricle, or formation of device-related thrombi are rare (<1%) complications of the procedure.

Transthoracic echocardiography is performed prior to discharge to confirm correct device position. Use of antibiotics during the intervention is commonplace, and prophylaxis against endocarditis is recommended for the few months until endothelization of the device. Full physical activity is possible as early as a few hours after the procedure. Follow-up treatment includes acetylsalicylic acid (100 mg q24h) with the addition of clopidogrel (75 mg q24h) for at least the first month. A follow-up TOE after 6 months showing closure of the PFO and no evidence of device-related thrombi signals cessation of antithrombotic treatment and endocarditis prophylaxis.

In the case of a relevant residual shunt, a follow-up (<5% of interventions using the Amplatzer PFO Occluder) repeat PFO closure can be considered. A residual shunt may be the consequence of an unstable device position, or due to the selection of too small a device at the first attempt, not covering all of the defect or only one of several defects (**4.35**). In occasional cases with a residual shunt after attempted PFO closure, there can be a second defect present (e.g. an atrial septal defect type II), not recognized during the initial TOE. The implantation of second closure device for any type of leaking is technically even less challenging than the first implantation procedure, due to the highly visible anatomical markers provided by the first device (**4.36–4.38**). In the authors' experience with more than 20 patients undergoing repeat PFO closure, no complications occurred during the second intervention or later at follow-up. Complete closure was achieved with the second intervention in 90% of patients.

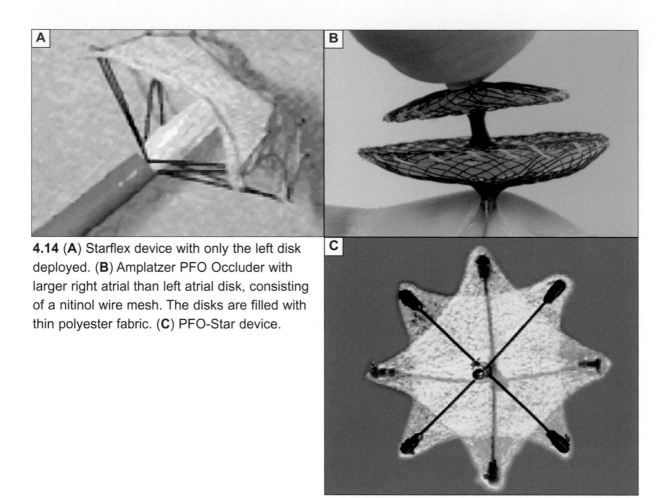

**4.14** (**A**) Starflex device with only the left disk deployed. (**B**) Amplatzer PFO Occluder with larger right atrial than left atrial disk, consisting of a nitinol wire mesh. The disks are filled with thin polyester fabric. (**C**) PFO-Star device.

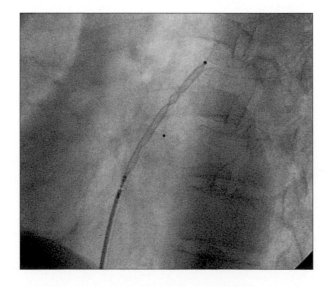

**4.15** Placement of an Amplatzer PFO Occluder. Step 1: the sheath is placed in the left atrium.

**4.16** Placement of an Amplatzer PFO Occluder. Step 2: after unfolding of the left atrial disk, the device is pulled against the septum primum.

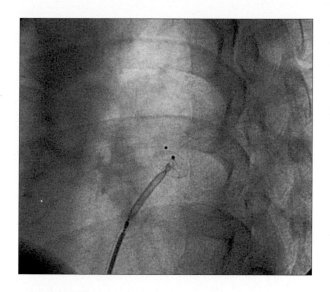

**4.17** Placement of an Amplatzer PFO Occluder. Step 3: the right atrial disk is unfolded in the right atrium.

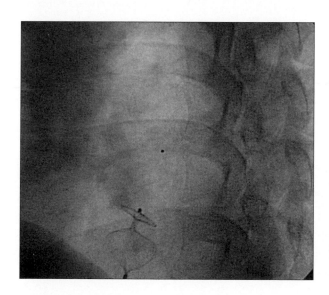

**4.18** Placement of an Amplatzer PFO Occluder. Step 4: the right-sided disk is pushed against the septum to flatten it and to ascertain stability.

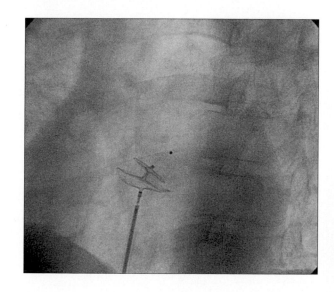

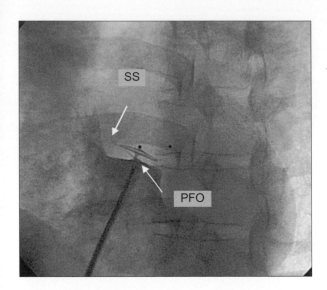

**4.19** Placement of an Amplatzer PFO Occluder. Step 5: correct device position is checked by manual right atrial dye injection. PFO: patent foramen ovale; SS: septum secundum.

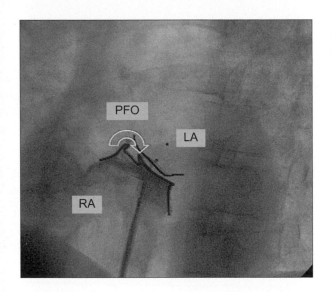

**4.20** Placement of an Amplatzer PFO Occluder. Step 5 (additional explanation): the septum secundum and the residual patency of the foramen ovale (curved arrow) can be identified to confirm device position. LA: left atrium; PFO: patent foramen ovale; RA: right atrium.

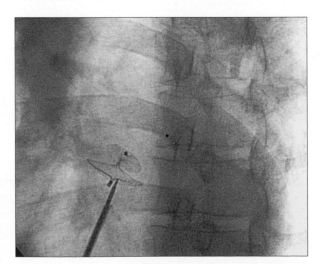

**4.21** Placement of an Amplatzer PFO Occluder. Step 6: the device is released (pusher unscrewed).

**4.22** Intracardiac ultrasound allows for continuous control of device position during the procedure, without the need for fluoroscopy. In contrast to transoesophageal echocardiography, there is no need for orotracheal intubation and general anaesthesia. However, intracardiac ultrasound devices are expensive as they are for single use only. LA: left atrium; RA: right atrium.

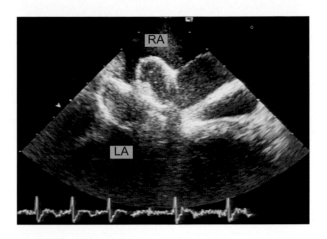

**4.23** The Pac-Man sign is a reliable marker for correct device position. The device appears to bite into the robust septum secundum at the upper left.

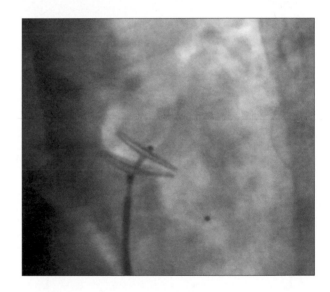

**4.24** The muscular septum secundum (yellow line) must be caught between the device disks (white line) straddling it and creating the Pac-Man sign.

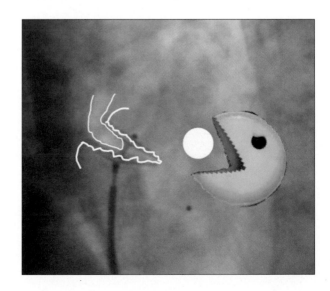

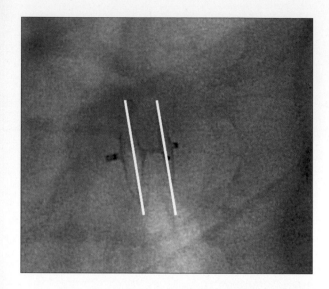

**4.25** Device placed in an atrial septal defect (ASD) of the septum primum (type II). Since the device fails to straddle the wedge-like thick septum secundum, no Pac-Man sign is seen.

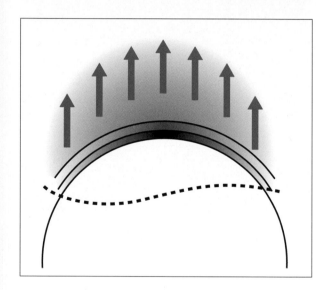

**4.26** Schematic diagram of a large foramen ovale seen from the left atrium.

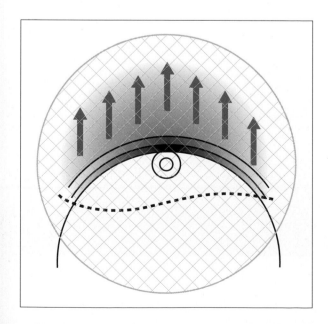

**4.27** Foramen of (**4.26**) after closure with an adequately sized and placed Amplatzer PFO occluder.

**4.28** Poor device position. The Pac-Man sign is not sufficiently present. The tip of the SS barely touches the rim of the device. A larger device is warranted. LA: left atrium; RA: right atrium; SP: septum primum; SS: septum secundum.

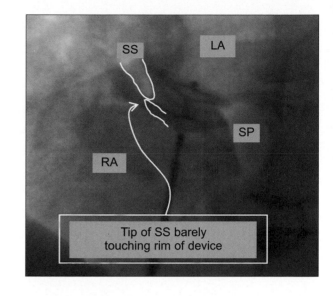

**4.29** A large occlusion device in relation to body size does not fit snugly. In addition, rubbing of the disks against the aorta may occur engendering a risk of erosion of the atrial wall. LA: left atrium; RA: right atrium.

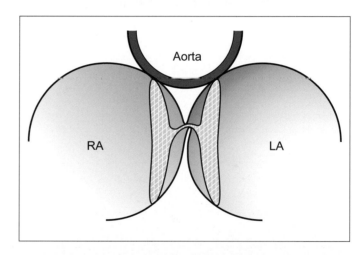

**4.30** The same situation as in (**4.29**) demonstrated by transoesophageal echocardiography. The dotted line delineates the right atrial disk indenting the aortic wall. LA: left atrium; RA: right atrium.

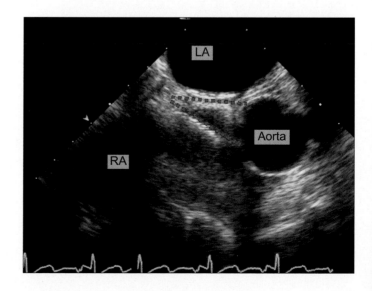

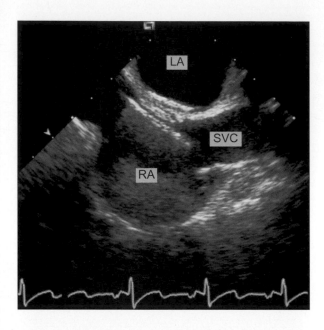

**4.31** As a further consequence of too large a device, the right atrial disk may partially protrude into the superior vena cava inflow tract. LA: left atrium; RA: right atrium; SVC: superior vena cava.

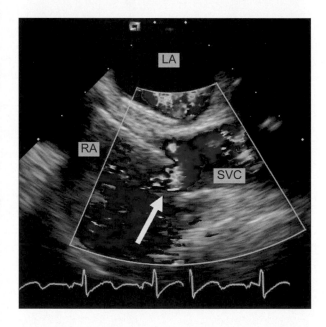

**4.32** The situation explained in (**4.31**) causes turbulent blood (arrow). LA: left atrium; RA: right atrium; SVC: superior vena cava.

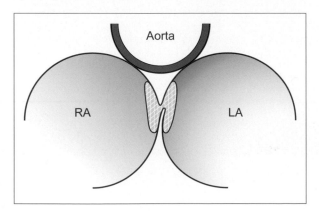

**4.33** The use of the smallest device with stable position and total covering of the defect is recommended. LA: left atrium; RA: right atrium.

**4.34** Transoesophageal echocardiography of a device (25 mm Amplatzer PFO occluder shown in the insert) 6 months after implantation. LA: left atrium; RA: right atrium; SVC: superior vena cava.

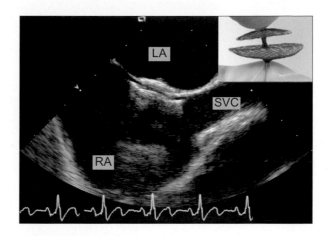

**4.35** Schematic diagram of a foramen ovale shunting only at the two angles. Two small Amplatzer PFO occluders are used preferably to one large one.

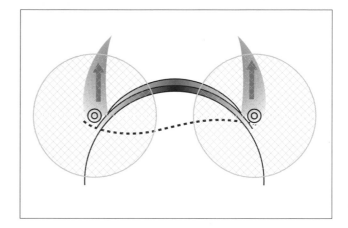

**4.36** In a patient with a residual shunt after a first closure attempt (PFO Star device), a second device is implanted to cover the residual defect. The catheter passes the residual defect and outlines the left atrium with contrast medium.

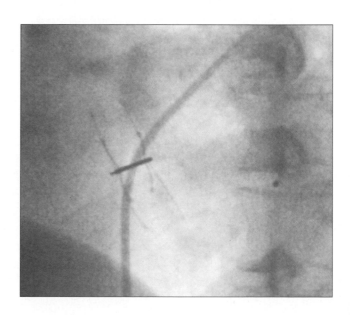

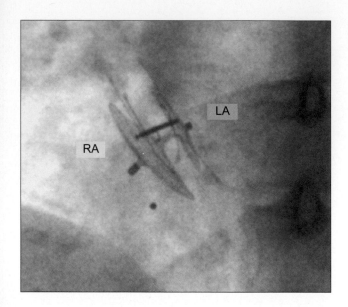

**4.37** The Amplatzer device straddling the leaky PFO Star of (**4.36**). LA: left atrium; RA: right atrium.

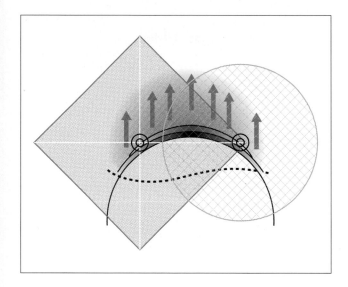

**4.38** The situation of (**4.36**) and (**4.37**) explained schematically.

## Conclusion

Only a decade after its first description, percutaneous closure of a PFO has become a common procedure in cardiac catheterization laboratories. Current indications for PFO closure include prevention of paradoxical embolism and correction of arterial desaturation in clinical settings with markedly elevated right atrial pressures, giving rise to a persistent right-to-left shunt. Clinical trials comparing the efficacy of interventional PFO closure versus medical treatment for prevention of paradoxical embolism are underway. For simplicity, speed, cost containment, and patient comfort, device implantation can be performed without the help of ultrasound. However, ascertaining correct device position on fluoroscopy before device release is mandatory. Newer device generations yield a complete closure rate of >90%, and a significant residual shunt rate of <5%. With the implantation of a second device in a further closure attempt in patients with a significant residual shunt, complete closure rate will be close to 100%. If TOE confirms PFO closure 6 months after the intervention, antiplatelet medication can be withdrawn if not otherwise indicated, and no further endocarditis prophylaxis is necessary for an endothelialized device.

# References

1 Hagen PT, Scholz DG, Edwards WD (1984). Incidence and size of patent foramen ovale during the first 10 decades of life: an autopsy study of 965 normal hearts. *Mayo Clin Proc,* **59**:17–20.

2 Agmon Y, Khandheria BK, Meissner I, *et al.* (1999). Frequency of atrial septal aneurysms in patients with cerebral ischemic events. *Circulation,* **99**:1942–1944.

3 Di Tullio M, Sacco RL, Venketasubramanian N, Sherman D, Mohr JP, Homma S (1993). Comparison of diagnostic techniques for the detection of a patent foramen ovale in stroke patients. *Stroke,* **24**:1020–1024.

4 De Marchi SF, Seiler C, Heule K, Aeschbacher BC (1998). Second harmonic imaging in transthoracic echocardiography for the diagnosis of a patent foramen ovale. *Schweiz Med Wochenschr,* **128**:45S (abstr).

5 Lechat P, Mas JL, Lascault G, *et al.* (1988). Prevalence of patent foramen ovale in patients with stroke. *N Engl J Med,* **318**:1148–1152.

6 Overell JR, Bone I, Lees KR (2000). Interatrial septal abnormalities and stroke: a meta-analysis of case-control studies. *Neurology,* **55**:1172–1119.

7 Homma S, Di Tullio M, Sacco RL (1998). Patent foramen ovale and stroke. In: *Stroke.* HJM Barnett, JP Mohr, BM Stein, FM Yatsu eds. Churchill Livingston Philadelphia, pp. 1013–1024.

8 Schuchlenz HW, Weihs W, Horner S, Quehenberger F (2000). The association between the diameter of a patent foramen ovale and the risk of embolic cerebrovascular events. *Am J Med,* **109**:456–462.

9 Windecker S, Wahl A, Chatterjee T, *et al.* (2000). Percutaneous closure of patent foramen ovale in patients with paradoxical embolism: long-term risk of recurrent thromboembolic events. *Circulation,* **101**:893–898.

10 Windecker S, Wahl A, Schwerzmann M, *et al.* (2002) Comparison of medical treatment with percutaneous closure of patent foramen ovale for secondary prevention of TIAs and strokes: a case control study. *J Am Coll Cardiol,* **39**:265A.

11 Wahl A, Meier B, Haxel B, *et al.* (2001). Prognosis after percutaneous closure of patent foramen ovale for paradoxical embolism. *Neurology,* **57**:1330–1332.

12 Homma S, Di Tullio MR, Sacco RL, Mihalatos D, Li Mandri G, Mohr JP (1994). Characteristics of patent foramen ovale associated with cryptogenic stroke. A biplane transesophageal echocardiographic study. *Stroke,* **25**:582–586.

13 Godart F, Rey C, Prat A, *et al.* (2000). Atrial right-to-left shunting causing severe hypoxaemia despite normal right-sided pressures. Report of 11 consecutive cases corrected by percutaneous closure. *Eur Heart J,* **21**:483–489.

14 Bansal RC, Marsa RJ, Holland D, Beehler C, Gold PM (1985). Severe hypoxemia due to shunting through a patent foramen ovale: a correctable complication of right ventricular infarction. *J Am Coll Cardiol,* **5**:188–192.

15 Konstantinides S, Geibel A, Kasper W, Olschewski M, Blumel L, Just H (1998). Patent foramen ovale is an important predictor of adverse outcome in patients with major pulmonary embolism. *Circulation,* **97**:1946–1951.

16 Schwerzmann M, Seller C, Lipp E, *et al.* (2001). Relation between directly detected patent foramen ovale and ischemic brain lesions in sport divers. *Ann Intern Med,* **134**:21–24.

17 Lipton RB, Stewart WF, Diamond S, Diamond ML, Reed M (2001). Prevalence and burden of migraine in the United States: data from the American Migraine Study II. *Headache,* **41**:646–657.

18 Del Sette M, Angeli S, Leandri M, *et al.* (1998). Migraine with aura and right-to-left shunt on transcranial Doppler: a case-control study. *Cerebrovasc Dis,* **8**:327–330.

19 Anzola GP, Magoni M, Guindani M, Rozzini L, Dalla Volta G (1999). Potential source of cerebral embolism in migraine with aura: a transcranial Doppler study. *Neurology,* **52**:1622–1625.

20 Lamy C, Giannesini C, Zuber M, *et al.* (2002). Clinical and imaging findings in cryptogenic stroke patients with and without patent foramen ovale: the PFO-ASA Study. Atrial Septal Aneurysm. *Stroke,* **33**:706–711.

21 Sztajzel R, Genoud D, Roth S, Mermillod B, Le Floch-Rohr J (2002). Patent foramen ovale, a possible cause of symptomatic migraine: a study of 74 patients with acute ischemic stroke. *Cerebrovasc Dis,* **13**:102–106.

22 Wilmshurst PT, Nightingale S, Walsh KP, Morrison WL (2000). Effect on migraine of closure of cardiac right-to-left shunts to prevent recurrence of decompression illness or stroke or for haemodynamic reasons. *Lancet,* **356**:1648–1651.

## Chapter 5

# Percutaneous Obliteration of Left Atrial Appendage in Atrial Fibrillation

*Stephan Windecker,* MD, *and*
*Bernhard Meier,* MD

## Introduction

Atrial fibrillation (AF) is the most common sustained cardiac arrhythmia and is a strong, independent risk factor for stroke and mortality. The incidence of the arrhythmia increases with age and affects approximately 5% of people at age 70 years and 10% of people >80 years of age[1]. Atrial fibrillation is responsible for 16% of all ischaemic strokes, with about two-thirds (10% of all ischaemic strokes) being cardioembolic, related to left atrial thrombi[2]. While rhythm control does not appear to reduce the risk of stroke, oral anticoagulation with vitamin K antagonists constitutes the mainstay of therapy. Vitamin K antagonist therapy reduces the stroke risk by 65% compared with placebo and by 45% compared with acetylsalicylic acid[1]. However, there is marked underuse of vitamin K antagonist therapy in patients with AF, related to the narrow therapeutic window, variability in pharmacokinetics, contraindications, and fear of bleeding complications (0.5% annual risk of cerebral haemorrhage).

## Left atrial appendage

The trabeculated left atrial appendage (LAA) is a remnant of the embryonic left atrium, whereas the smooth walled left atrial cavity is formed by the outgrowth of the pulmonary veins. The LAA is lined by endothelium and contains pectinate muscles which run largely parallel to each other and give rise to the trabeculated surface[3]. The LAA lies antero-laterally in the left atrioventricular sulcus, and is in close contact with the pulmonary artery superiorly and the left ventricular free wall inferiorly. The anatomy of the LAA is rather complex, with a windsock-like configuration, consisting of multiple lobes and a narrow junction, which is connected to the left atrium (**5.1–5.3**)[4, 5]. The size of the LAA varies considerably, with an orifice measuring 5–27 mm in diameter and a LAA length measuring 16–51 mm. Quantification of atrial natriuretic factor (ANF) from excised atrial appendages revealed a content of approximately 30% of all cardiac ANF. The LAA has a distinct pattern of contraction: Doppler flow measurements reveal a quadriphasic pattern. The LAA has been considered a decompression chamber at times of increased atrial pressure due to its high distensibility, the anatomical location high in the left atrium, and the ability to secrete ANF.

Atrial fibrillation not only affects remodelling of the proper left atrium but also of the LAA. Thus, LAA casts of patients with AF have been found more voluminous, with larger orifices and fewer branches compared to patients in normal sinus rhythm. In addition, lower appendage Doppler flow velocities and LAA ejection fraction have been observed in patients with AF. These pathological changes result in stasis and predispose to thrombus formation within the LAA cavity (**5.4**, **5.5**). Of note, transoesophageal echocardiographic studies revealed that >90% of all thrombi related to AF originate from the LAA[6]. Unfortunately, strokes related to LAA thrombus embolism are larger and more disabling compared to strokes of other aetiology, presumably related to the relatively large thrombus size nested within the LAA cavity.

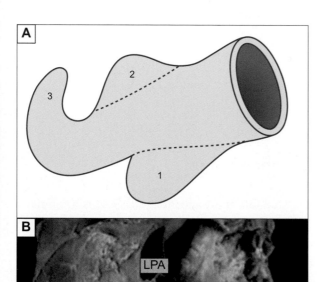

**5.1** Schematic diagram (**A**) of left atrial appendage (LAA) with typical windsock-like appearance and multiple lobes (1—3). Anatomical specimen (**B**) of LAA with two lobes as viewed from outside. LA: left atrium; LIPV: left inferior pulmonary vein; LPA: left pulmonary artery; LSPV: left superior pulmonary vein. (Courtesy of Veinot et al.[4])

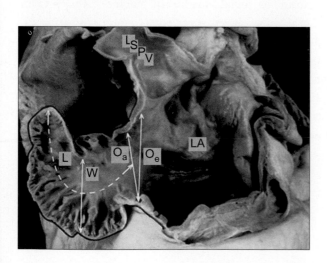

**5.2** Anatomical specimen of left atrial appendage (LAA) as viewed when opened from the left atrium. Note the landmarks for anatomical and echocardiographic measurements of the LAA. Oe: echocardiographic orifice; Oa: anatomic orifice; L: length; W: width; LA: left atrium; LSPV: left superior pulmonary vein. (Courtesy of Veinot et al.[4])

**5.3** Left atrial appendage cast and its shadow from an autopsy specimen revealing the complex anatomy, with multiple bends, a windsock-like appearance, and take-off multiple small branches. These small branches (white arrows) were not visible on transoesophageal echocardiography. (Courtesy of Stöllberger *et al.* [5])

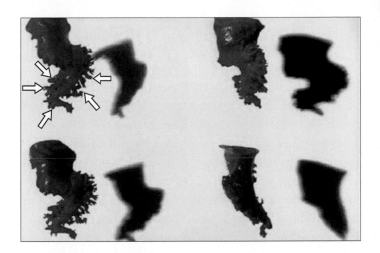

**5.4** Transoesophageal echocardiography of left atrial appendage (LAA) revealing a thrombus attached to the LAA wall in a patient with atrial fibrillation.

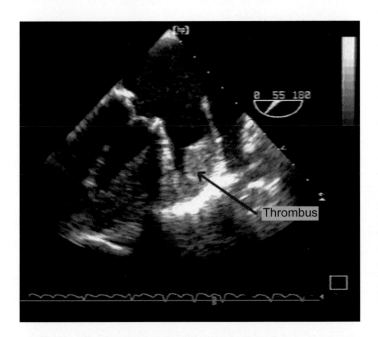

**5.5** Virtual angioscopic view of left atrial appendage (LAA) showing an embolus in motion and the trabeculated surface and complex LAA anatomy with multiple lobes and bends. (Courtesy of AstraZeneca.)

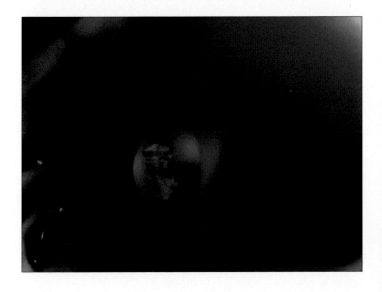

## Percutaneous obliteration of the left atrial appendage

The pivotal observation that the vast majority (90%) of thrombi related to stroke in patients with AF originate from the LAA, stirred the therapeutic interest to obliterate the LAA as a means of stroke prophylaxis in patients with AF[6]. Indeed, it has become common practice to remove the LAA at the time of mitral valve surgery, and it is also a routine part of the surgical maze procedure in patients with atrial fibrillation. Currently, a randomized clinical trial is examining the potential of surgical LAA amputation to reduce stroke risk in patients undergoing heart surgery who are at high risk of developing AF[7].

Recently, a dedicated device for LAA obliteration via the percutaneous route was introduced. The percutaneous left atrial appendage occluder (PLAATO[TM]) system (**5.6**) consists of a nitinol metal cage with multiple outwardly bent anchors covered by a polytetrafluoroethylene (PTFE) membrane, and a delivery catheter, which houses the restrained implant[8].

The implantation procedure uses a femoral venous puncture followed by trans-septal access to the left atrium using routine technique. The trans-septal sheath is exchanged for the delivery catheter (11 French), which is used to perform an angiogram of the LAA to determine the implant size, either directly or guided by a diagnostic catheter. Following placement of the delivery catheter within the LAA, the implant is positioned by withdrawal of the catheter from the LAA (and active opening of the device in case of the PLAATO technique). The implant position is checked by a series of criteria including effective occlusion of the LAA by the device, a residual compression (>10%) of the device, and a 'wiggling' manoeuvre (**5.7**)[9]. Device embolization is prevented by careful assessment of the above release criteria, oversizing the implant relative to the measured parameters by 20–40%, and by the anchors on the implant surface. In case of unsatisfactory results the device is fully retrievable and can be collapsed in the delivery sheath for another placement attempt. Animal studies revealed complete LAA occlusion, no evidence for thrombi on the implant surface, and complete healing 3 months after device implantation (**5.8**, **5.9**).

The clinical performance of the device has been investigated in a recent study of 87 patients with AF, and at least one high risk feature for embolic stroke and a contraindication for treatment with vitamin K antagonists (Sievert H, personal communication). Patients received acetylsalicylic acid indefinitely and clopidogrel for a duration of 6 months. The procedure was successful in 86 (99%) patients and complicated by hemopericardium in 6 (8%) patients. During follow-up two deaths, one minor stroke, two transient ischaemic attacks, and three gastro-intestinal bleeds were observed.

The ease of use of the Amplatzer device for closure of patent foramen ovale and atrial septal defects has led to the investigation of the Amplatzer technique for percutaneous obliteration of the LAA (**5.10**). Following trans-septal puncture, a LAA angiogram is performed to determine size and anatomy. Thereafter, the Amplatzer introducer sheath (7–9 French) is positioned in the LAA and an Amplatzer septal occluder is introduced, with a neck a few millimetres smaller than the orifice of the LAA. The left disk of the device is deployed in the LAA by withdrawal of the delivery sheath, and the right disk is then released and usually placed at the LAA entrance. The position is verified by a left atrial angiogram through the delivery sheath, assessment of device configuration, and a 'wiggle' test during which the distal part of the device should remain stable. Then the device is released by unscrewing from the delivery cable (**5.11**).

Percutaneous LAA obliteration using the Amplatzer technique has been reported in 16 patients with AF, at high risk for stroke, and with a contraindication for therapy with vitamin K antagonist[10]. The procedure was successful in 15 (94%) patients and complicated by device embolization in one patient. During follow-up of 5 patient years, no device-related complications or embolic events were noted. In addition, the LAA was occluded in all successfully treated patients without evidence of thrombosis at the atrial side of the device (**5.12**).

**5.6** PLAATO implant consisting of a nitinol metal cage with outward bent anchors and covered with ePTFE. PLAATO: percutaneous left atrial appendage transcatheter occluder; LA: left atrium; LAA: left atrial appendage; ePTFE: expanded polytetrafluoroethylene. (Courtesy of Nakai et al.[8])

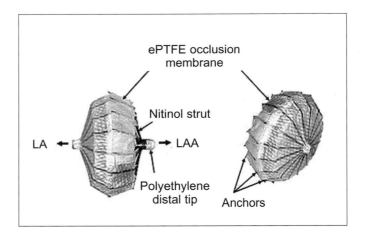

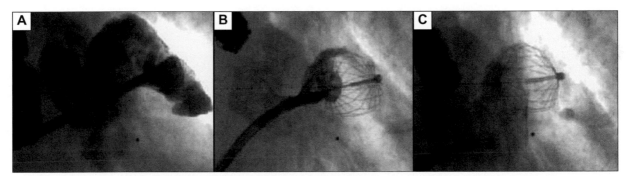

**5.7** Angiographic left atrial appendage appearance before (**A**), during (**B**), and after (**C**) percutaneous left atrial appendage transcatheter occluder (PLAATO) implantation.

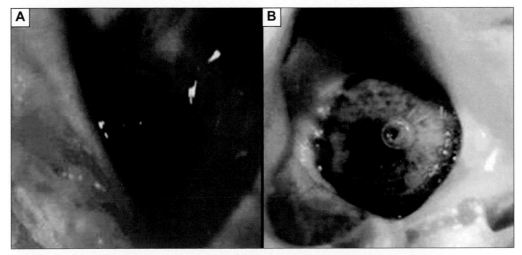

**5.8** Anatomical specimen of left atrial appendage with percutaneous device (PLAATO) 1 month (left) and 3 months (right) after implantation in dogs. Note the snug fit of the implant and the endothelialization of the device surface. (Courtesy of Nakai et al.[8])

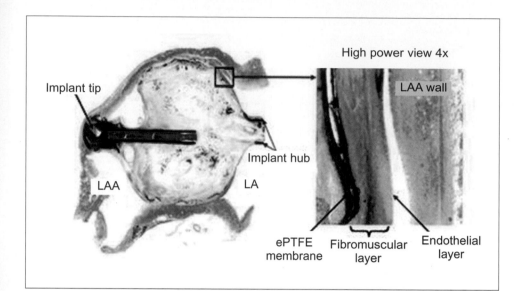

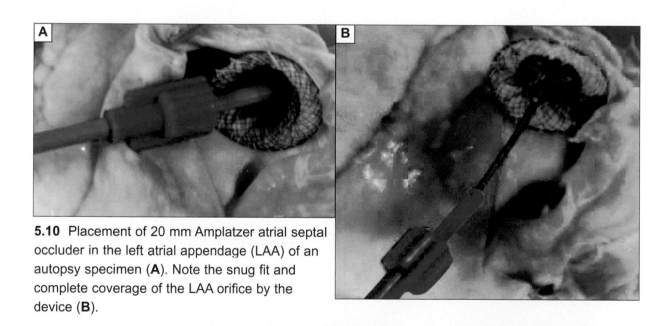

**5.9** Light microscopic specimen 3 months after PLAATO implantation in a dog. Note the device apposition against the LAA endocardial surface without evidence of residual gaps. LA: left atrium; LAA: left atrial appendage; ePTFE: expanded polytetrafluoroethylene; PLAATO: percutaneous left atrial appendage transcatheter occluder. (Courtesy of Nakai et al.[8])

**5.10** Placement of 20 mm Amplatzer atrial septal occluder in the left atrial appendage (LAA) of an autopsy specimen (**A**). Note the snug fit and complete coverage of the LAA orifice by the device (**B**).

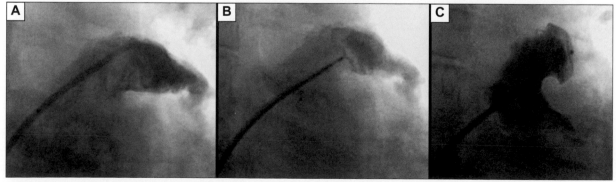

**5.11** Angiography (antero-posterior view) of left atrial appendage before (**A**), during (**B**), and after implantation (**C**) of a 20 mm Amplatzer atrial septal occluder in a 67-year-old patient with atrial fibrillation and increased risk of bleeding due to Osler s disease.

**5.12** Transoesophageal echocardiography 3 months after implantation of a 9 mm Amplatzer atrial septal occluder in left atrial appendage (LAA) in a patient with atrial fibrillation. Note the snug device position, the complete exclusion of the LAA by the device, and the absence of thrombus on the atrial site of the device.

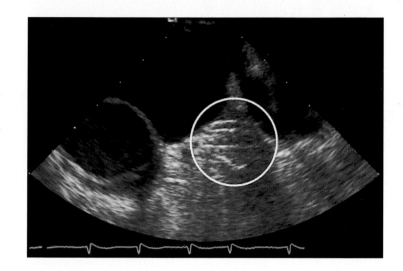

## Conclusion

Percutaneous LAA obliteration has been shown to be feasible in patients with AF, using the LAA dedicated PLAATO device and the Amplatzer septal occluder. They can be easily combined with other therapeutic catheter procedures such as closure of a patent foramen ovale or an atrial septal defect, mitral balloon valvuloplasty, coronary angioplasty, or ablation for AF. The incidence of complications appears acceptable in this population who are at high risk of stroke and have contraindications for vitamin K antagonist therapy.

Future studies will elucidate the mid- and long-term safety and efficacy of percutaneous LAA obliteration. The results of such studies will have to compare favourably with medical treatment with vitamin K antagonists or the novel direct oral thrombin inhibitor ximelagatran in preventing thromboembolism in patients with AF.

## References

1  Hart RG, Halperin JL, Pearce LA, *et al.* (2003). Lessons from the Stroke Prevention in Atrial Fibrillation trials. *Ann Intern Med*, **138**:831–838.

2  Hart RG, Halperin JL (2001). Atrial fibrillation and stroke: concepts and controversies. *Stroke*, **32**: 803–808.

3  Al-Saady NM, Obel OA, Camm AJ (1999). Left atrial appendage: structure, function, and role in thromboembolism. *Heart*, **82**:547–554.

4  Veinot JP, Harrity PJ, Gentile F, *et al.* (1997). Anatomy of the normal left atrial appendage: a quantitative study of age-related changes in 500 autopsy hearts: implications for echocardigraphic examination. *Circulation*, **96**:3112–3115.

5  Stöllberger, Ernst G, Bonner E, *et al.* (2003). Left atrial appendage morphology: comparison of transesophageal images and postmortem casts. *Z Kardiol*, **92**:303–308.

6  Blackshear JL, Odell JA (1996). Appendage obliteration to reduce stroke in cardiac surgical patients with atrial fibrillation. *Ann Thorac Surg*, **61**:755–759.

7  Crystal E, Lamy A, Connolly SE, *et al.* (2003). Left Atrial Appendage Occlusion Study (LAAOS): a randomized clinical trial of left atrial appendage occlusion during routine coronary bypass surgery for long-term stroke prevention. *Am Heart J*, **145**:174–178.

8  Nakai T, Lesh MD, Gerstenfeld EP, *et al.* (2002). Percutaneous left atrial appendage occlusion (PLAATO) for preventing cardioembolism. *Circulation*, **105**:2217–2222.

9  Sievert H, Lesh MD, Trepels T, *et al.* (2002). Percutaneous left atrial appendage transcatheter occlusion to prevent stroke in high-risk patients with atrial fibrillation: early clinical experience. *Circulation*, **105**: 1887–1889.

10 Meier B, Palacios IF, Windecker S, *et al.* (2003). Transcatheter left atrial appendage occlusion with Amplatzer devices to obviate anticoagulation in patients with atrial fibrillation. *Catheter Cardiovasc Interv*, **60**:417–422.

# Catheter Ablation of Supraventricular and Ventricular Tachycardias

*Etienne Delacrétaz, MD, and Jürg Fuhrer, MD*

## Introduction

In this chapter, current approaches for ablation of a broad spectrum of cardiac arrhythmias are presented. In order to limit technical information and for didactic purposes, material obtained using only one multisite mapping system (CARTO®) is presented, although other interesting systems are available.

Advances in catheter ablation therapy have led to a widespread increase in its use in management of cardiac arrhythmias. Catheter ablation can be defined as the use of an electrode catheter to destroy small areas of myocardial tissue or conduction system, or both, that are critical to the initiation and/or maintenance of cardiac arrhythmias. During radiofrequency (RF) ablation, current flows into the tissue in contact with the electrode in alternating direction at high frequency. Thermal injury is the principal mechanism of tissue destruction during RF catheter ablation procedures (**6.30, 6.31**).

For most types of supraventricular arrhythmias, medical treatment with antiarrhythmic drugs is not completely effective. In addition, antiarrhythmic drugs can be associated with a number of side-effects. The high success rates and low complication rates of catheter ablation have revolutionized treatment of such conditions as Wolff–Parkinson–White syndrome and atrioventricular (AV) nodal re-entrant tachycardia[1] (**6.1–6.4**). More recently, catheter ablation has become the first-line therapy for treatment of patients with atrial flutter and focal or re-entry atrial tachycardia[1] (**6.6–6.20**). Incisional atrial tachycardia is mediated by macro-re-entry around the scar of a prior surgical atriotomy (**6.14–6.20**). These tachycardias, frequently seen as late sequelae after surgical repair of congenital heart disease, can also be treated with RF ablation with high success rates[2]. The most recent developments in ablative therapy relate to interventional treatment of atrial fibrillation (**6.24–6.29**).

Paroxysmal atrial fibrillation can be cured by catheter ablation in selected patients[3].

In addition, catheter ablation is a useful treatment for selected patients with ventricular tachycardia (VT)[3, 4] (**6.32–6.40**). It should be considered for patients with recurrent, symptomatic idiopathic ventricular tachycardia (**6.37–6.40**) and is the first-line treatment for bundle branch re-entry ventricular tachycardia[4]. However, the majority of sustained monomorphic VTs are caused by re-entry involving a region of ventricular scar (**6.32, 6.33**). The scar is most commonly caused by an old myocardial infarction. Because of the risk of sudden cardiac death in patients with VT and structural heart disease, the first-line therapy is implantation of a defibrillator. Ablation therapy can decrease frequent episodes of post-infarct VT causing recurrent therapies from an implanted defibrillator, and can be lifesaving for patients with incessant VT[4].

As the spectrum of ablatable arrhythmias has broadened, the ablation procedures have, in some cases, become technically challenging. In many situations, visualization of the catheter tip in relation to the cardiac anatomy is crucial. Several new technologies have provided means for non-fluoroscopic tracking of catheter tip position and orientation in three-dimensional space (**6.13, 6.15–6.20, 6.33, 6.36, 6.39–6.40**). Newly developed multielectrode catheters or multisite mapping systems allow delineation of complex re-entry arrhythmias in relation to the anatomy of atrial or ventricular scar or incisions[4]. Successful ablation of a large atrial or ventricular re-entrant circuit is achieved either by targeting an isthmus where the circuit can be interrupted with a small number of RF lesions, or by creating a line of RF lesions through a region containing the re-entry circuit.

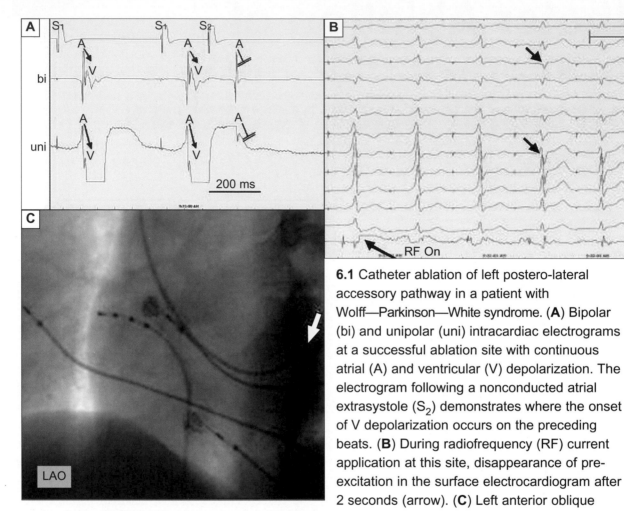

**6.1** Catheter ablation of left postero-lateral accessory pathway in a patient with Wolff—Parkinson—White syndrome. (**A**) Bipolar (bi) and unipolar (uni) intracardiac electrograms at a successful ablation site with continuous atrial (A) and ventricular (V) depolarization. The electrogram following a nonconducted atrial extrasystole (S$_2$) demonstrates where the onset of V depolarization occurs on the preceding beats. (**B**) During radiofrequency (RF) current application at this site, disappearance of pre-excitation in the surface electrocardiogram after 2 seconds (arrow). (**C**) Left anterior oblique (LAO) view of the ablation catheter positioned at the atrioventricular sulcus laterally via retrograde approach across the aortic valve (arrow).

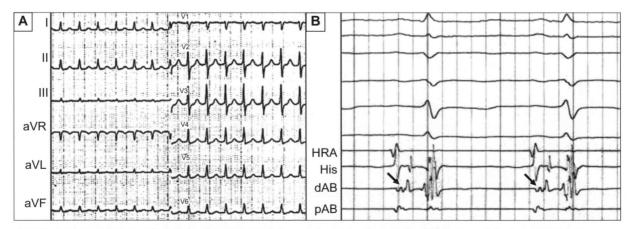

**6.2** Catheter ablation of atrioventricular nodal re-entrant tachycardia (**A**) can safely be achieved based on well established criteria. Intracardiac recordings on the right panel (**B**) are high right atrium (HRA), His, distal and proximal ablation catheter (dAB and pAB). The slow potential is of low amplitude, rounded, sometimes double hump-shaped (arrows).

**6.3** Slow pathway potential is a sharp deflection occurring 10—40 msec after the local atrial potential (arrows). Radiofrequency ablation at this site usually results in transient accelerated junctional rhythm. Intracardiac recordings are high right atrium (HRA), His, distal and proximal ablation catheter (dAB and pAB).

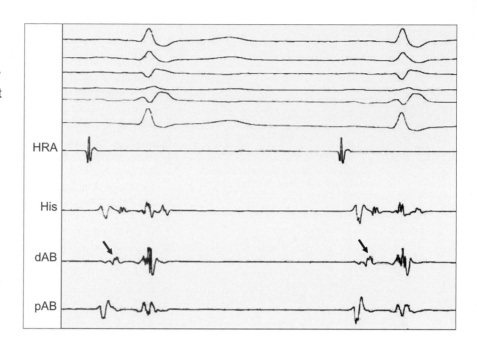

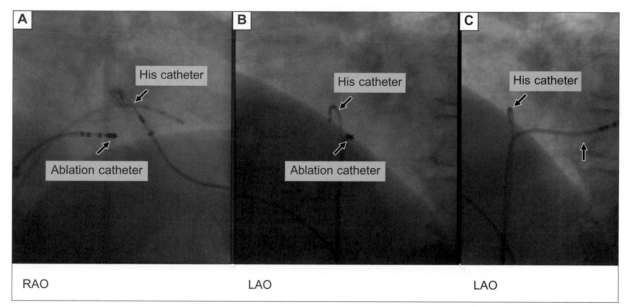

**6.4** Fluoroscopic right anterior oblique (RAO) and left anterior oblique (LAO) (**A**, **B**) views of catheter position during radiofrequency ablation of atrioventricular nodal re-entrant tachycardia. The His catheter is positioned to record a proximal and distal His electrogram at the anterior aspect of the septum. The ablation catheter is positioned to record a slow pathway potential (caudally to the coronary sinus ostium). Note on the LAO view that the ablation catheter is directed toward the septum (clockwise torque). (**C**) A catheter has been introduced in the coronary sinus (arrow) to show its anatomical position.

**New classification of atrial tachyarrhythmias**

Classification into *flutter* or *tachycardia* depending on the *rate* and presence of a stable baseline on the ECG is obsolete

*Substrate: slow conduction and unidirectional conduction block*

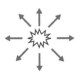

*Mechanism: triggered activity or automaticity*

• *Macro-re-entrant atrial tachycardias*

Macro-re-entry around normal structures (terminal crest, eustachian ridge) or around atrial lesions:
— Isthmus-dependent atrial flutter (counterclockwise and clockwise)
— Incisional atrial tachycardia
— Left atrial flutter

• *Focal atrial tachycardias*

Radial spread of activation

**6.5** New classification of atrial tachyarrhythmias, according to the mechanism (either macro-re-entry or focal activity). The classification into flutter or tachycardia depending on the rate and presence of stable baseline is obsolete. ECG: electrocardiogram.

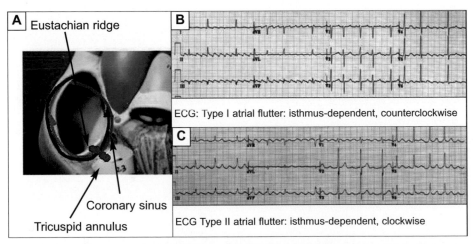

**6.6** Isthmus-dependent atrial flutter. (**B**) Typical atrial flutter is characterized in the 12-lead electrocardiogram (ECG) by saw-toothed deflections in the inferior leads (II, III, and avF), and positive deflections in V1. The right atrial activation during typical atrial flutter is counterclockwise (left panel, blue arrow), spreading from the septum to the roof of the right atrium and from the roof to the lateral free wall. (**C**) ECG with reversed typical flutter with positive flutter waves in the inferior leads and negative deflections in V1. The right atrial activation (**A**, red arrow) during reverse typical atrial flutter is clockwise. Red dots represent sites to be targeted with radiofrequency ablation to create isthmus block and to abolish atrial flutter.

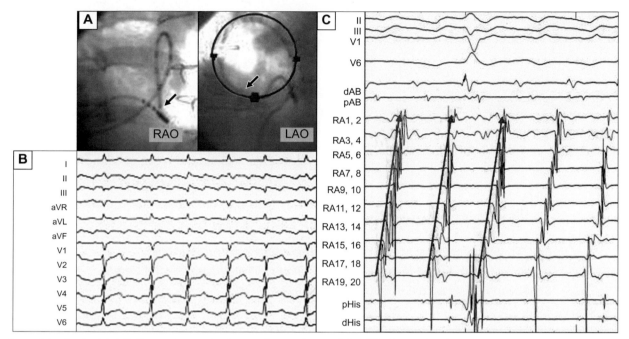

**6.7** Mapping of typical atrial flutter using a dodecapolar catheter (Halo□) shown in right anterior oblique (RAO) and left anterior oblique (LAO) projections (**A**). The distal electrode 1 is at the tip of the catheter (black arrow). The ablation catheter is positioned medially at the ventricular side of the cavo-tricuspid isthmus. (**B**) 12-lead electrocardiogram showing typical atrial flutter. (**C**) During typical atrial flutter, right atrial activation spreads along the Halo catheter from the proximal electrode pairs (RA19, 20, close to the coronary sinus ostium) towards the distal electrode pairs (RA1, 2, red arrows).

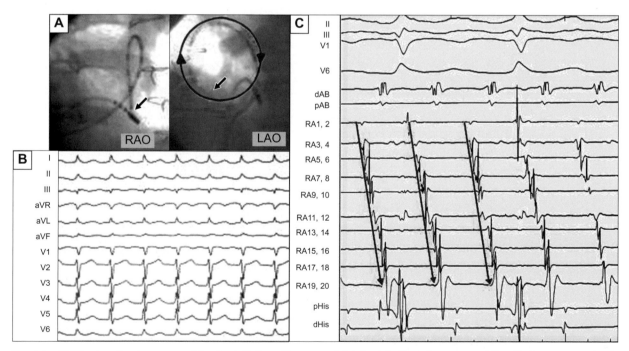

**6.8** The patient in (**6.7**) also had reversed typical flutter. Reversed typical flutter shows positive flutter waves in the inferior leads and negative deflections in V1. (**B**) The right atrial activation sequence during reversed typical atrial flutter is clockwise (**A**: left anterior oblique (LAO) view, red arrow), spreading from the lateral free wall to the atrial roof and from the roof to the septum. (**C**) During reverse typical atrial flutter, right atrial activation spreads along the Halo catheter from the distal electrode pairs (RA1, 2) towards the proximal electrode pairs (RA19, 20, red arrows). Both atrial flutters were abolished by radiofrequency ablation of the cavo-tricuspid isthmus. RAO: right anterior oblique.

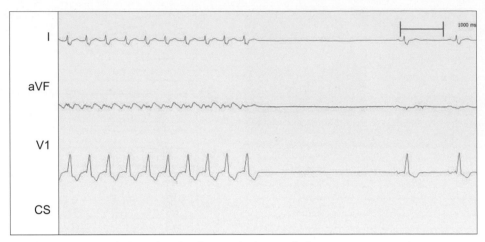

**6.9** Termination of typical atrial flutter during radiofrequency current application at the cavo-tricuspid isthmus. Sinus activity resumes following a 3.6 second offset pause. CS: coronary sinus.

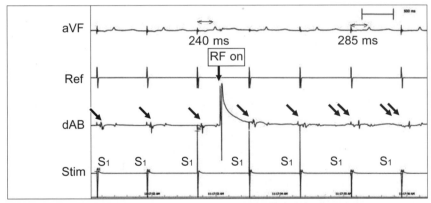

**6.10** Mapping and ablation of typical and reversed typical atrial flutter can be performed with two quadripolar catheters during atrial flutter or during sinus rhythm. The elimination of residual conduction through the cavo-tricuspid isthmus is depicted in the figure. The ablation catheter (dAb) is positioned at the cavo-tricuspid isthmus, the stimulation catheter (Stim and Ref) is located in the low right atrium. Before elimination of residual conduction, a centre potential is registered (arrows) during stimulation from the low right atrium. Residual conduction is eliminated 1.5 seconds after radiofrequency (RF) current is turned on, with sudden appearance of a double potential with an isoelectric interval of 160 ms, indicating isthmus block (double arrows). Simultaneously, the interval from stimulus to QRS is prolonged from 240 ms to 285 ms, due to the altered activation of the right atrium.

**6.11** In this example, the pacing catheter is positioned in the coronary sinus. The ablation catheter is positioned at the lateral aspect of the cavo-tricuspid isthmus. During stimulation from the coronary sinus, the activation wavefront (red arrow) travels towards the right atrium and activation of the medial aspect of the isthmus can be recorded by the ablation catheter (A). Following radiofrequency ablation, conduction through the isthmus is blocked, and activation of the lateral aspect of the isthmus is delayed (A ), occurring after activation of the posterior or superior right atrium (green arrow). CS: coronary sinus; OS: ostium; LAO: left anterior oblique.

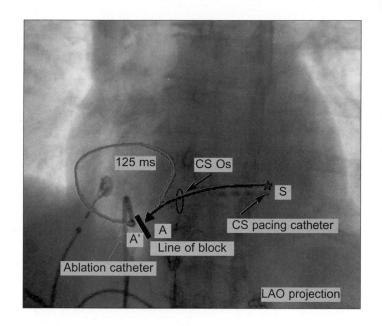

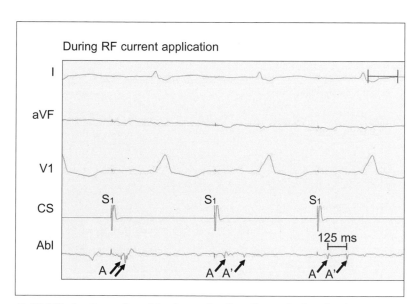

**6.12** Elimination of residual conduction through the Cosio isthmus as shown by pacing from coronary sinus during radiofrequency ablation of atrial flutter. The atrial activation recorded by the ablation catheter following the first stimulus ($S_1$) (on the left) shows a relatively complex electrogram (central potential). Following the next stimulus during radiofrequency current application, appearance of a widely spread double potential (A and A') occurs, indicating isthmus block. The first atrial deflection (A) represents activation of the septal aspect of isthmus, whereas the second atrial deflection (A') represents activation of the lateral aspect of the isthmus, occuring 125 ms later and following activation of the posterior or superior right atrium.

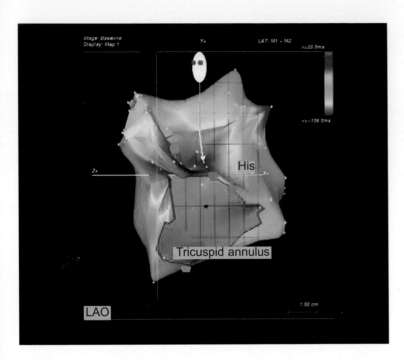

**6.13** Catheter ablation of focal, right atrial tachycardia. Electroanatomical mapping using CARTO™ system: Activation map of the right atrium during tachycardia, in left anterior oblique (LAO) view. The tricuspid annulus is represented in brown. The activation time is colour-coded and the time scale for colour-coding is indicated in the bar at the upper right. Red indicates the earliest depolarization at the origin of the tachycardia, close to the tricuspid annulus, at 12:00 o clock (arrow). Yellow, green, and blue indicate subsequent radial spread of the depolarization wavefront. Application of radiofrequency current at the earliest site (arrow) abolished atrial tachycardia. Yellow dots show sites where a His deflection was recorded.

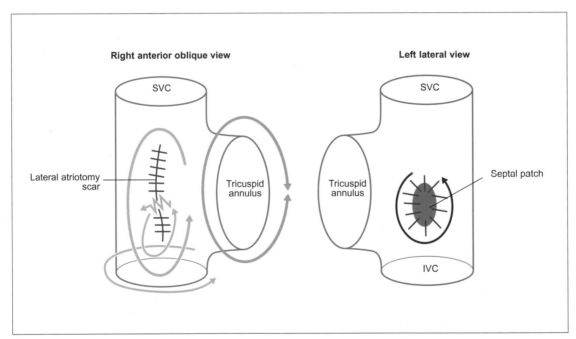

**6.14** Diagram depicting the right atrium and different intra-atrial re-entrant tachycardia circuits late after surgical repair of congenital heart disease. In green, typical and reverse typical atrial flutter (isthmus dependent). In yellow, incisional atrial tachycardia related to the lateral atriotomy scar. In red, re-entry around a septal patch. SVC: superior vena cava; IVC: inferior vena cava.

**6.15** Electroanatomic mapping of typical atrial flutter. Left panel: Activation map of the right atrium in left anterior oblique (LAO) view during counterclockwise, isthmus-dependent, atrial flutter occurring late after repair of atrial septum defect. The depolarization wave travels around the tricuspid annulus (TA, in brown), in a counterclockwise direction. The activation time is colour-coded: the red areas denote sites of early activation, followed by yellow, green, and blue. IVC: inferior vena cava. Right panels: Bottom view of the cavo-tricuspid isthmus with red dots representing radiofrequency lesions forming a line of conduction block across the cavo-tricuspid isthmus.

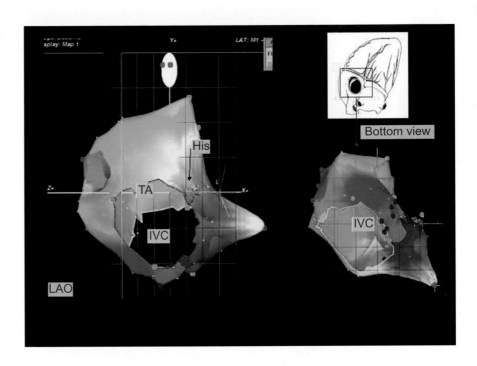

**6.16** Propagation maps of reversed typical atrial flutter demonstrating the depolarization wavefront (red) in a left anterior oblique view travelling around the tricuspid annulus. Grey areas in the lateral atrium represent unexcitable scar related to previous atriotomy, characterized by very low voltage electrograms. The four frames (**A–D**) represent the temporal propagation of activation throughout the flutter cycle. Areas in red represent depolarization within a 30 ms time frame. From the exit of the cavo-tricuspid isthmus (**A**), a broad proportion of the lateral right atrium depolarizes very quickly towards the roof of the right atrium (**B**). The re-entry wave circles in a clockwise direction and depolarizes the septum (**C**) before it reaches the entrance of the isthmus (**D**). Red dots demonstrate radiofrequency current lesions at the septal aspect of the cavo-tricuspid isthmus, abolishing atrial flutter.

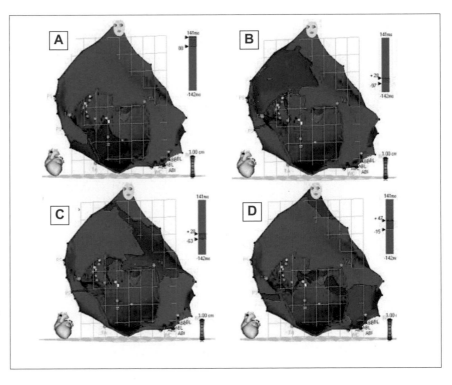

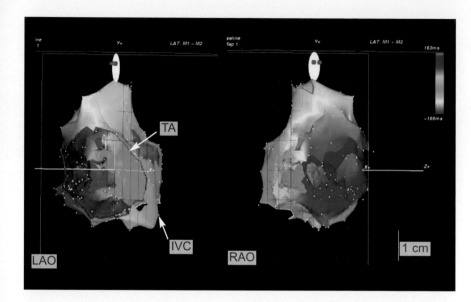

**6.17** Electroanatomic mapping of slow reverse typical atrial flutter in a patient with dilated right atrium, late after surgical repair of atrial septal defect. The activation wavefront propagates around the tricuspid annulus (TA, in brown), in a clockwise direction. The activation time is colour-coded: the red areas denote sites of early activation, followed by yellow, green, blue, and purple. The grey areas denote the atriotomy scar and the septal patch. IVC: inferior vena cava; LAO: left anterior oblique; RAO: right anterior oblique.

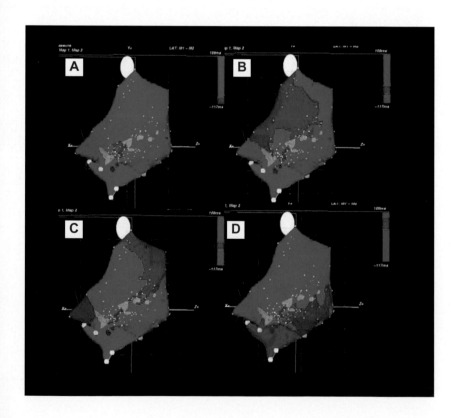

**6.18** Propagation maps of re-entrant atrial tachycardia demonstrating a depolarization wavefront (red) in a right posterior oblique (RPO) view. Grey areas in the lateral atrium represent unexcitable scar related to previous atriotomy, characterized by very low voltage electrograms. The four frames (**A–D**) represent the temporal propagation of activation throughout the macro-re-entrant circuit cycle. Areas in red represent depolarization within a 30 ms time frame. From the exit of this narrow pathway formed by the scar (**A**), a broad proportion of the postero-superior right atrium depolarizes very quickly (**B**). The re-entry waves then circle superiorly in a clockwise direction and inferiorly in a counterclockwise direction (**C**), colliding with the inferior aspect of the scar (**D**).

**6.19** Activation sequence map of the right atrium during tachycardia in the patient in (**6.18**) (posterior oblique view). The activation time is colour-coded (bar, upper right): the red areas denote sites of early activation, and purple denotes the latest activation. During tachycardia, the depolarization wave travels from the mid-posterior right atrium superiorly. The superior (clockwise) wavefront returns to the region proximal to the exit site (purple) to complete the circuit by propagating through a narrow isthmus bounded by two areas of unexcitable scar (in grey). Two radiofrequency lesions, indicated by the red tags, extending between two scarred areas were created. Tachycardia terminated during the second radiofrequency lesion. The line transecting the isthmus was then completed with three additional lesions.

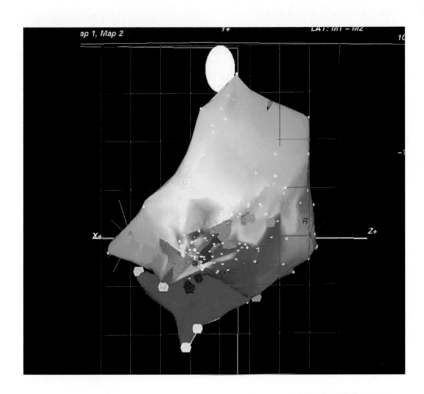

**6.20** Propagation maps of re-entrant atrial tachycardia demonstrating a depolarization wavefront (red) in a right anterior oblique view. Grey areas in the low lateral atrium represent unexcitable scar related to previous atriotomy, characterized by very low voltage electrograms. The four panels (**A–D**) represent the temporal propagation of electrical activation throughout the macro-re-entrant circuit cycle. Areas in red represent depolarization within a 30 ms time frame. From the exit of the conduction isthmus delineated by the scar and the inferior vena cava (**A**), a broad proportion of the postero-superior right atrium depolarizes very quickly (**B**, **C**). The re-entry waves then circle superiorly in the clockwise direction, re-entering the tachycardia isthmus (**D**).

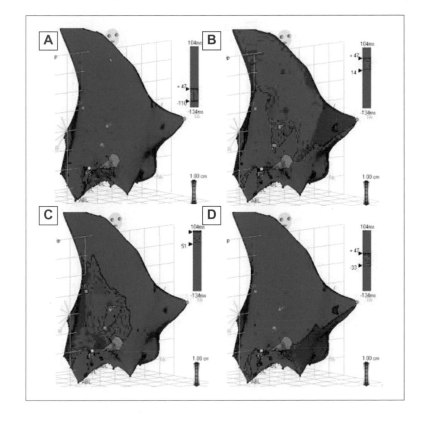

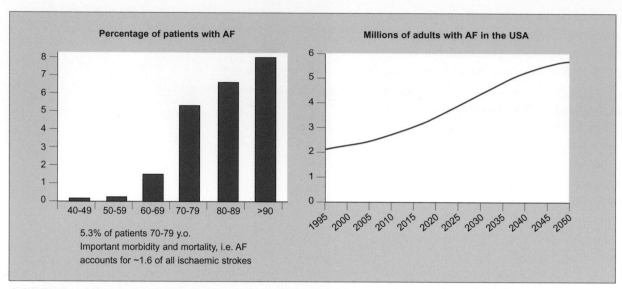

**6.21** Epidemiology of atrial fibrillation (AF). In the next 30 years, the number of adults with paroxysmal, persistent, or permanent atrial fibrillation may double[5].

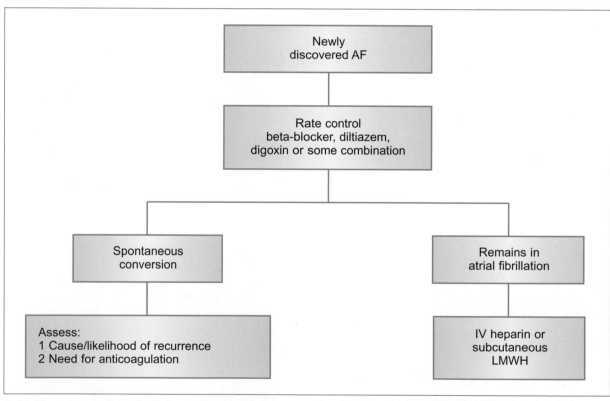

**6.22** First steps of treatment of newly diagnosed atrial fibrillation (AF). According to the guidelines of the American Heart Association, the American College of Cardiology, and the European Society of Cardiology, subcutaneous low molecular weight heparin (LMWH) can replace intravenous heparin.

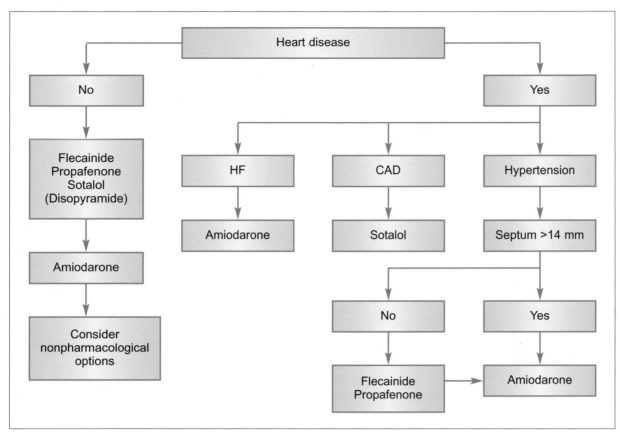

**6.23** Selection of anti-arrhythmic drug for rhythm control according to underlying heart disease (according to the American Heart Association, the American College of Cardiology, and the European Society of Cardiology). CAD: coronary artery disease; HF: heart failure

**6.24** Rhythm strip showing focal atrial fibrillation: Focal ectopic activity with P on T in bigeminy (arrows) triggering atrial fibrillation. Most of the ectopic beats are not conducted to the ventricles.

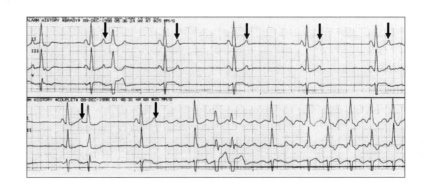

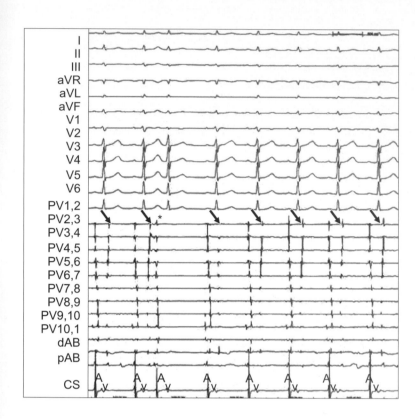

**6.25** Concealed pulmonary vein activity in a patient with focal atrial fibrillation. PV1, 2—PV10, 1 are recordings from a decapolar Lasso® catheter, mapping the circumference of pulmonary vein and demonstrating pulmonary vein concealed ectopy in bigeminy (arrows). Due to the short coupling intervals the left atrium is refractory. Only the second pulmonary vein ectopic beat (with a slightly longer coupling interval) is conducted to the atria (*), with a single supraventricular ectopic beat in surface electrocardiogram ( P on T ). dAb and pAb: recordings from the ablation catheter in the same pulmonary vein; CS: coronary sinus electrogram showing atrial (A) and ventricular (V) activity of the left cavities.

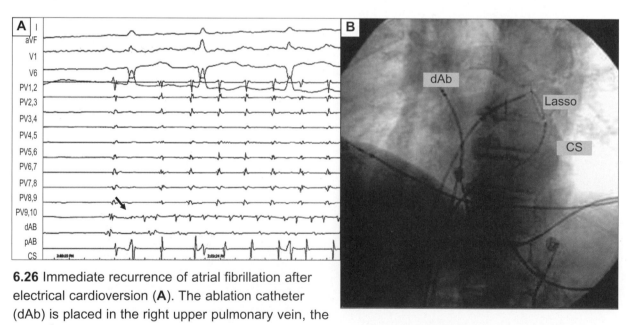

**6.26** Immediate recurrence of atrial fibrillation after electrical cardioversion (**A**). The ablation catheter (dAb) is placed in the right upper pulmonary vein, the Lasso® catheter in the left upper pulmonary vein, and a quadripolar catheter in the coronary sinus (CS) (**B**). Pulmonary vein activity triggers atrial fibrillation. The earliest pulmonary vein activity can be registered by the ablation catheter in the right upper pulmonary vein (arrow), consistent with an arrhythmogenic focus in this vein.

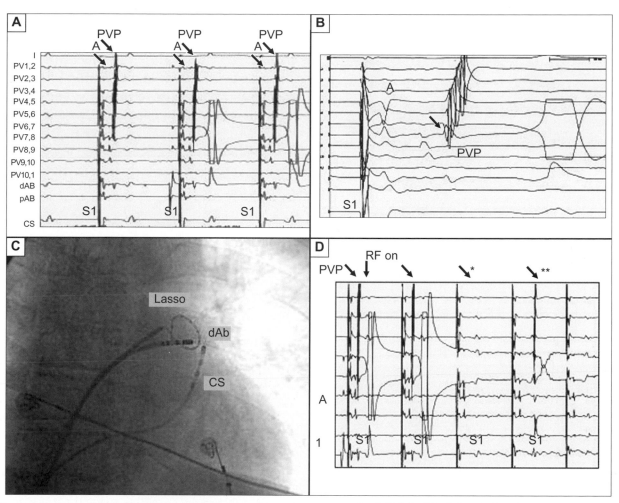

**6.27** Ablation of focal atrial fibrillation in the left superior pulmonary vein (LSPV). (**A**) Stimulation in the coronary sinus (S1) allows separation of the pulmonary venous potentials (PVP, arrows) from atrial far field recordings (A) in LSPV. (**B**) Circumferential mapping of the pulmonary venous orifice allows detection of earliest local activation between PV6, 7 and PV7, 8 (arrow). (**C**) The ablation catheter (dAb) is positioned at the site of earliest PV activation. There is also a catheter in the coronary sinus (CS). (**D**) Radiofrequency (RF) current application at this site immediately interrupts the connection between left atrium and LSPV (missing PVP, *). Subsequently, focal pulmonary vein activity resumes, dissociated from the paced atrial activity (**).

**6.28** Ablation of focal atrial fibrillation in the right superior pulmonary vein. Following initial dissection of a first bridging connection between the left atrium and the pulmonary vein, successive atrial (A) and pulmonary vein activation (PVP) can easily be demonstrated. The earliest local pulmonary vein activation can be recorded by the ablation catheter (dAb). Delivery of radiofrequency (RF) current at this site disconnects the last muscle bridge (*), with block of conduction to the pulmonary vein (missing PVP).

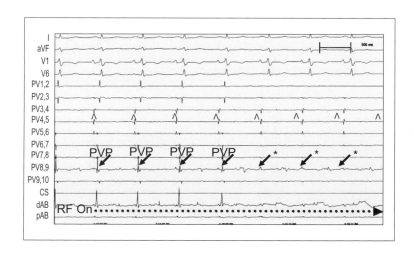

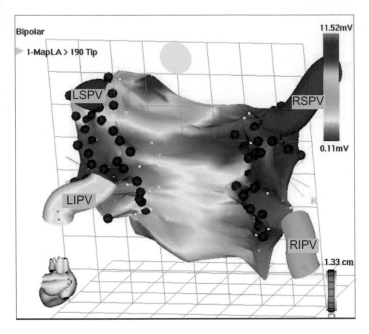

**6.29** Anatomic approach for catheter ablation of atrial fibrillation. A voltage map of the left atrium in a posterior view is shown. The bipolar voltage of the local electrograms is colour-coded (low voltage in red). RSPV, RIPV, LSPV, LIPV: right superior, right inferior, left superior, and left inferior pulmonary veins. After localization of the four pulmonary veins, encircling of their four ostia with radiofrequency lesions is performed, to insulate electrically the triggers within the pulmonary veins and around the pulmonary vein ostia from the rest of the left atrium.

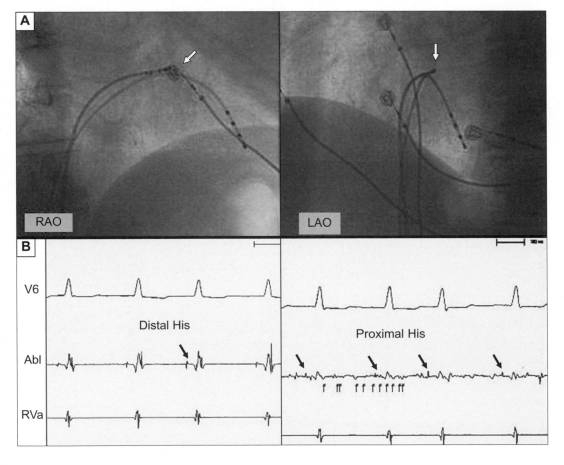

**6.30** Catheter ablation of the atrioventricular junction in a patient with permanent atrial fibrillation with rapid ventricular rate refractory to drug therapy. (**A**) The extremity of the ablation catheter (arrows) is positioned at the antero-septal aspect of the atrioventricular groove to record a His deflection. (**B**) Recording of a distal His deflection. The catheter is slightly withdrawn to record a proximal His deflection (right panel), together with atrial fibrillation waves (f). LAO: left anterior oblique; RAO: right anterior oblique.

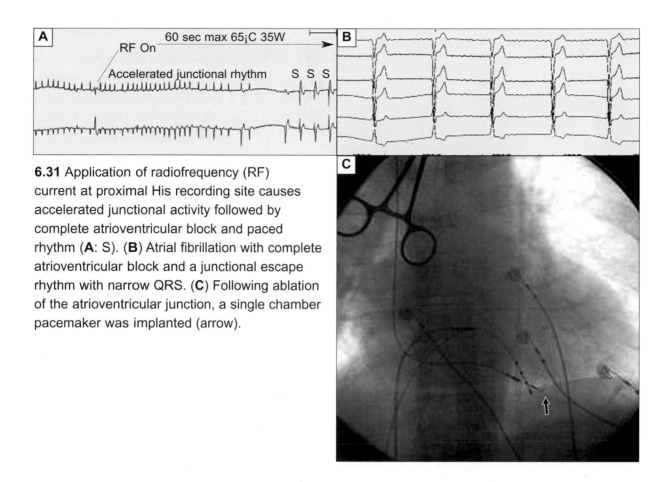

**6.31** Application of radiofrequency (RF) current at proximal His recording site causes accelerated junctional activity followed by complete atrioventricular block and paced rhythm (**A**: S). (**B**) Atrial fibrillation with complete atrioventricular block and a junctional escape rhythm with narrow QRS. (**C**) Following ablation of the atrioventricular junction, a single chamber pacemaker was implanted (arrow).

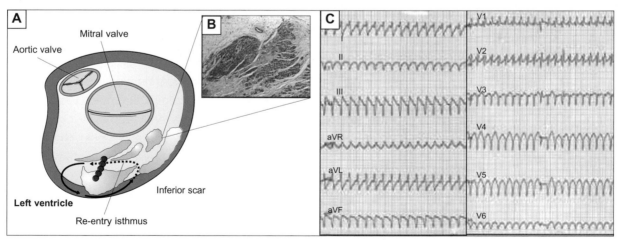

**6.32** Ablation of monomorphic ventricular tachycardia late after myocardial infarction (**C**). The majority of sustained monomorphic ventricular tachycardias are caused by re-entry involving a region of ventricular scar (**A**). The scar is most commonly caused by an old myocardial infarction. (**B**) Fibrosis between surviving myocyte bundles decreases cell-to-cell coupling, causing slow conduction, which promotes re-entry. These re-entry circuits often contain a narrow isthmus of abnormal conduction which can be targeted with radiofrequency ablation (**A**, red dots transecting the re-entry isthmus). However, the critical parts of the circuit may be difficult to localize, rendering catheter ablation challenging. Recently, electroanatomic mapping of tachycardia was shown to be effective for ablation of scar-related ventricular tachycardias.

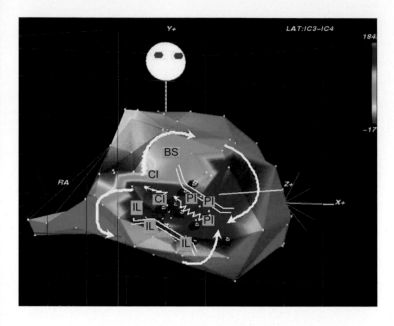

**6.33** Electroanatomic mapping for ablation of ventricular tachycardia. Activation map of the left ventricle during ventricular tachycardia. The left ventricle is shown in right anterior oblique view. The colours indicate the activation sequence and arrows have been drawn to clarify the spread of the depolarization wavefront. The re-entry circuit is located in the septum. The wavefront starts at the red area (exit) near the base of the septum and splits into two loops that circle around the superior and inferior aspect of the septum toward the apex, re-entering the circuit isthmus. Double lines indicate zone of functional or anatomical block. Re-entry circuit sites may be classified by entrainment mapping (CI: central isthmus site; PI: proximal isthmus site; BS: bystander site; IL: inner loop site). Isthmus sites (proximal, central, or exit sites) are ablation targets. Red dots indicate radiofrequency ablation lesions at proximal and central isthmus sites which terminated ventricular tachycardia.

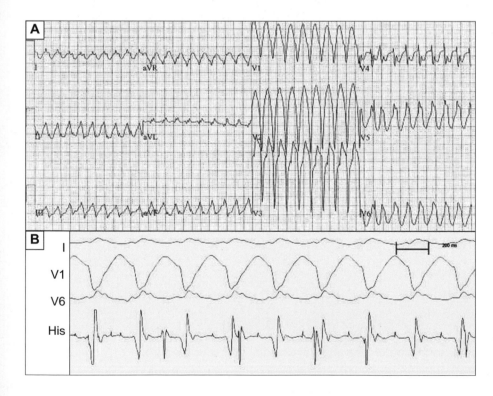

**6.34** A patient with dilated cardiomyopathy presented with palpitations. Twelve-lead electrocardiogram showed monomorphic wide QRS tachycardia, with a left bundle branch block morphology at a rate of 210 bpm. Since QRS complexes during tachycardia were identical to those during sinus rhythm, bundle branch re-entry tachycardia was suspected. The differential diagnosis included supraventricular tachycardia with left bundle branch block. The electrophysiological study showed inducible ventricular tachycardia during isoproterenol infusion, with a cycle length of 300 ms and a QRS morphology identical to that of clinical ventricular tachycardia. During ventricular tachycardia, an H deflection (depolarization of His bundle) preceded each QRS by 80 ms, consistent with bundle branch re-entry tachycardia (**B**).

**6.35** Bundle branch re-entry tachycardia occurs in patients with nonischaemic cardiomyopathies, mostly valvular heart disease and dilatative cardiomyopathy, and can be successfully abolished with catheter ablation of the right bundle branch. (**A**) The ablation catheter (Abl) is positioned to record a right bundle (RB) branch electrogram. Since the patient has left bundle branch block, radiofrequency ablation of the right bundle branch produces complete heart block after a short burst of activity of the right bundle branch (**B**), and ventricular pacing is initiated (S). (**C**) Re-entry circuit during bundle branch re-entry tachycardia. The depolarization propagates down the right bundle branch, through the interventricular septum, and back to the His bundle via the left bundle branch. Ablation of the right bundle branch interrupts the circuit.

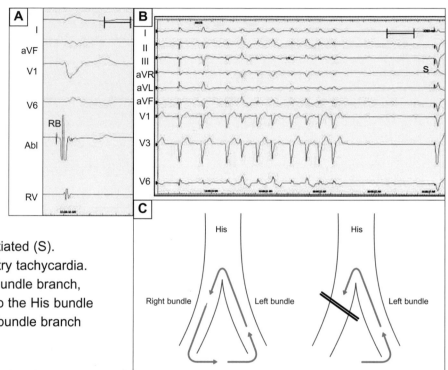

**6.36** Ventricular tachycardia in a patient late after surgical repair of congenital heart disease. In patients with Fallot tetralogy, intra-operative mapping studies demonstrated a re-entry around the ventriculotomy scar, in clockwise or counterclockwise directions (**A**). Red dots represent how radiofrequency lesions can be created to interrupt tachycardia. (**B**) Ventricular tachycardia in a patient with transposition of the great vessels late after Rastelli operation. Recurrent ventricular tachycardia triggered frequent shocks from an implantable defibrillator. In the electrophysiology laboratory, two ventricular tachycardia morphologies were inducible (VT-1 and VT-2), consistent with re-entry in a clockwise and counterclockwise direction

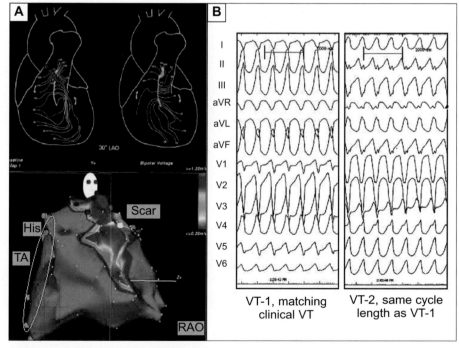

around the scar. Since ventricular tachycardia was haemodynamically poorly tolerated, ablation was guided by sinus rhythm substrate mapping (left lower panel). The right ventricle is represented in right anterior oblique view. Areas with normal electrocardiogram voltage are represented in purple and blue. Red and yellow colours represent sites with low voltage electrogram (below 0.5 mV) consistent with scar. TA: tricuspid annulus. A line of radiofrequency lesions was created between the scar and a pulmonary conduit to interrupt re-entry tachycardia.

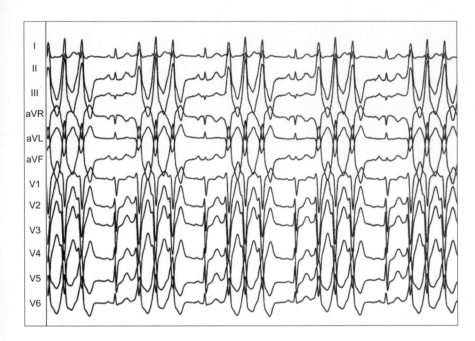

**6.37** Twelve-lead electrocardiogram of repetitive nonsustained ventricular outflow tract tachycardia. QRS complexes show high amplitude R wave in inferior leads. Precordial transition zone is >V4. Monomorphic ventricular tachycardia (VT) in patients without structural heart disease is referred to as idiopathic and has a focal origin. The most common idiopathic VT originates from a focus in the outflow tract of the right ventricle. Tachycardia may occur in repetitive bursts or in sustained VT. In some patients, VT and frequent premature beats are severely symptomatic and warrant treatment. These VT can be abolished by catheter ablation in most of the patients.

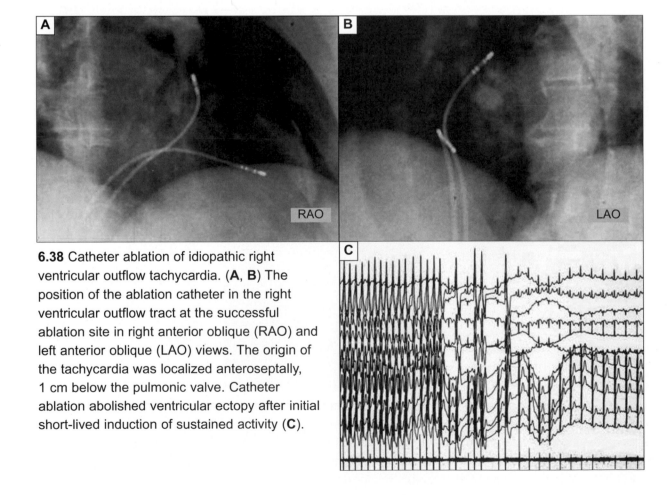

**6.38** Catheter ablation of idiopathic right ventricular outflow tachycardia. (**A**, **B**) The position of the ablation catheter in the right ventricular outflow tract at the successful ablation site in right anterior oblique (RAO) and left anterior oblique (LAO) views. The origin of the tachycardia was localized anteroseptally, 1 cm below the pulmonic valve. Catheter ablation abolished ventricular ectopy after initial short-lived induction of sustained activity (**C**).

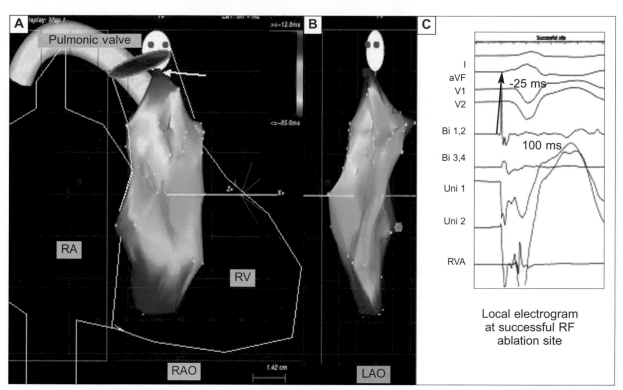

**6.39** Catheter ablation of idiopathic right ventricular tachycardia. (**A, B**) Electroanatomical mapping of right ventricular outflow tract during tachycardia. Mapping of the rest of the right ventricle was not performed. The activation time is colour-coded (bar, upper right). Red indicates the earliest depolarization at the origin of the tachycardia, close to the pulmonic valve. Yellow, green, and blue indicate subsequent radial spread of the depolarization wavefront. Application of radiofrequency current at the earliest site (arrow) abolished ventricular tachycardia. A yellow dot shows the site where a His deflection was recorded. LAO: left anterior oblique; RA: right atrium; RAO: right anterior oblique; RV: right ventricle. (**C**) The timing of the local bipolar (Bi1,2) electrogram 25 ms earlier than the QRS onset, as well as the typical QS morphology of the unipolar electrogram (Uni1) at the site of origin, where radiofrequency (RF) ablation successfully abolished tachycardia.

**6.40** Propagation maps showing activation of the right ventricular outflow tract during ventricular tachycardia, demonstrating the focal origin of the excitation at the postero-septal aspect of the outflow tract and the rapid radial spread of the activation wavefront (red) in right anterior oblique (RAO) view of the outflow tract (the rest of the right ventricle was not depicted). Red represents depolarized areas within a 6—10 ms time frame. LO: location only (at these sites in contact with the pulmonic valve, no electrical activity could be registered).

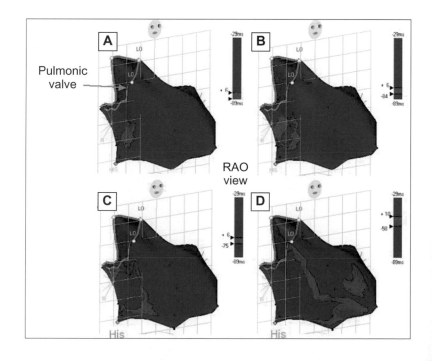

## Conclusion

The majority of arrhythmias can potentially be cured with catheter ablation therapy. The safety and efficacy of catheter ablation for treatment of AV nodal re-entrant tachycardia, Wolff–Parkinson–White syndrome, focal atrial tachycardia, atrial flutter, and idiopathic VT is well established. Catheter ablation for treatment of atrial fibrillation and VT secondary to structural heart disease remains an area of active research.

## References

1 Calkins H (2001). Radiofrequency catheter ablation of supraventricular arrhythmias. *Heart*, **85**:594–600.

2 Delacrétaz E, Ganz LI, Soejima K, *et al.* (2001). Multi atrial macro-re-entry circuits in adults with repaired congenital heart disease: entrainment mapping combined with three-dimensional electroanatomic mapping. *J Am Coll Cardiol*, **37**(6):1665–1676.

3 Lin D, Marchlinski FE (2003). Advances in ablation therapy for complex arrhythmias: atrial fibrillation and ventricular tachycardia. *Curr Cardiol Reports*, **5**(5):407–414.

4 Delacrétaz E, Stevenson WG (2000). Catheter ablation of ventricular tachycardia. *Heart*, **84**(5):553–559.

5 Go AS, Hylek EM, Phillips KA, *et al.* (2002). Prevalence of diagnosed atrial fibrillation in adults: national implications for rhythm management and stroke prevention: the anticoagulation and risk factors atrial fibrillation (ATRIA) study. *JAMA*, **285**(18):2370–2375.

# Chapter 7

# Implantation of Cardioverter-Defibrillator

*Nicola Schwick,* MD

## Introduction

Sudden cardiac death is one of the great challenges in electrophysiology. The best therapeutic option in preventing ventricular tachyarrhythmias leading to sudden death is the implantation of an automatic cardioverter-defibrillator. Since the first automatic defibrillator was successfully implanted in 1980 in a human being[1], the devices have gradually improved in technology and size.

## Device technology

Starting with abdominal devices and epicardial patches that required thoracotomy for implantation, today's technology offers small devices that can be implanted subcutaneously with endocardial or subcutaneous electrodes implanted under local anaesthesia. The latest models of the implantable cardioverter-defibrillator (ICD) are not only easy to implant but also offer additional options, including multisite pacing or cardioversion of atrial flutter and atrial fibrillation.

Although every ICD can apply defibrillation shocks (up to 40 J), several other options are available to treat ventricular tachycardias which do not require immediate cardioversion. The physician can choose between several modes of overdrive pacing and features to distinguish ventricular from supraventricular tachyarrhythmias. The newer models of ICDs are conceived to facilitate an individual and safe programming, but some pitfalls persist (*Table 7.1*).

Another big advantage of the new generation ICD is the storage of intracardiac electrocardiograms which help the physician to evaluate the treatment of the ICD.

Although the ICD can be life-saving, side-effects have to be taken into account. The perioperative mortality rate with transvenous leads and subcutaneous or subpectoral device is <1%. Adverse events are described in up to 50% of patients with a transvenous ICD system[2] (*Table 7.2*). However, use of ICDs for more than 20 years has led to continuously increasing safety and also new indications.

## Indications

According to the current guidelines[3–6] not only secondary prevention but also primary prevention of sudden cardiac death is a target of ICD. The guidelines are continuously being adapted according to medical evidence. A summarized flow chart can be seen below (**7.1**). Continuous effort is being put into improving the technology and to prove the cost effectiveness of ICDs.

**Table 7.1 Discrimination features for supraventricular tachycardias**

| Feature | Meaning | Problems |
|---|---|---|
| Onset (%, ms) | • VTs are supposed to begin with a sudden rise of heart rate in contrast to ST. | • SVTs may begin suddenly.<br>• Exercise-induced VTs do not have a sudden onset. |
| Stability (%, ms) | • VTs are supposed to be regular in contrast to atrial fibrillation. | • SVT and ST can also be regular.<br>• Polymorph VT can be irregular. |
| Morphology | • VTs are supposed to have a different (e.g. wider) QRS-complex than ST or SVT. | • Intermittent bundle branch block can change QRS morphology.<br>• Some features are dependant on the patient s position. |
| Relation of atrial and ventricular signals (only for dual chamber devices) | • Ventricular signals faster than atrial signals mean a ventricular-atrial dissociation and support the diagnosis of VT.<br>• Atrial signals faster than ventricular signals support the diagnosis of atrial flutter or atrial fibrillation. | • 1:1 sensing of ventricular and atrial signals may occur in VT with retrograde AV-node conduction and in SVT, and therefore has to be further discriminated. This discrimination can be affected by antiarrhythmic agents which can slow AV-node conduction.<br>• Atrial undersensing can appear in atrial fibrillation.<br>• Atrial lead dislocation may affect algorithms. |

AV: atrioventricular; ST: sinus tachycardia; SVT: supraventricular tachycardia; VT: ventricular tachycardia.

**Table 7.2 Adverse events of ICD therapy**

| ICD- procedure related | ICD-related (nonprocedural) |
|---|---|
| Infection/sepsis | DFT rise, pacing threshold rise |
| Haemodynamic compromise | Sensing problems: undersensing or T-wave oversensing |
| RV perforation with pericardial effusion/tamponade | Lead-specific problems (e.g. isolation problems, lead fracture) |
| Pneumothorax/haemothorax | Inappropriate shocks due to SVT or ST |
| Perforation of subcutaneous leads | |
| Lead dislodgement | |
| Device dislodgement | |
| Pain, arm mobility reduction | |
| Lead connection problems | |
| Thromboembolism/thrombosis | |
| Procedure-induced arrhythmia | |

DFT: Defibrillation threshold; RV: right ventricle; ST: sinus tachycardia; SVT: supraventricular tachycardia

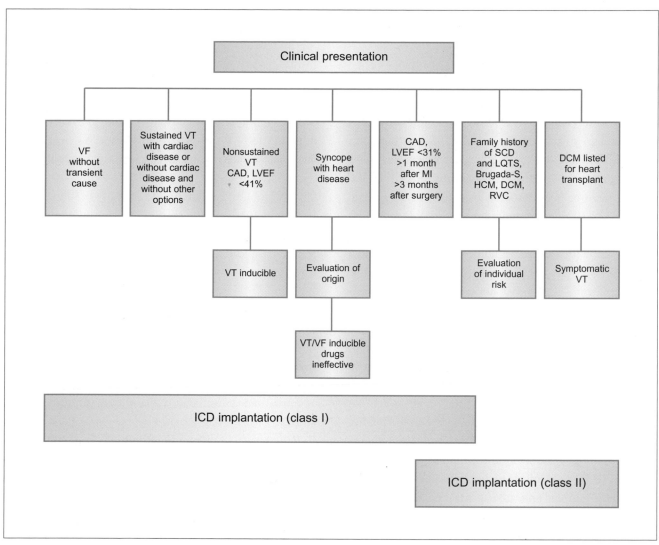

**7.1** Indications for implantation of an implantable cardioverter-defibrillator (ICD). The indications according to the guidelines of European Society of Cardiology (ESC) and American College of Cardiology (ACC) are indicated here. Consider that in some patients both class I and class II indications are possible, and further investigation is necessary. There are slight differences between the ESC and ACC recommendations. Brugada-S: Brugada syndrome; CAD: coronary artery disease; DCM: dilated cardiomyopathy; HCM: hypertrophic cardiomyopathy; LQTS: long-QT syndrome; LVEF: left ventricular ejection fraction; MI: myocardial infarction; RVC: right ventricular cardiomyopathy; SCD: sudden cardiac death; VF: ventricular fibrillation; VT: ventricular tachycardia.

## Implantation technique

Today the ICD is implanted like a pacemaker in the awake patient, in an operating room or catheterization laboratory. Lead placement is achieved via the prepared cephalic vein or puncture of the subclavian vein into the right ventricle, atrium, coronary sinus, or vena cava. Sometimes an additional defibrillation lead is necessary to achieve sufficient defibrillation thresholds. This can either be placed in the superior vena cava or subcutaneously in the inferior dorsal thorax. The active device is usually implanted below the left clavicle, either subpectorally or subcutaneously. This configuration leads to good defibrillation thresholds in most of the cases. If necessary, right-sided implantations are also possible. In children, abdominal implantation with a non-active device and additional defibrillation leads (intra-venously and subcutaneously) may be necessary.

Intra-operative testing for defibrillation threshold (DFT) is mandatory, in spite of a certain risk of complications as ventricular fibrillation has to be induced. The induction of ventricular fibrillation can easily be achieved via the ICD, either using low energy shocks in the vulnerable T-wave phase or by applying a 50 Hz burst. The DFT has to be at least 10 J beneath the maximum defibrillation output of the device. If the device is implanted under local anaesthesia, deep sedation or general anaesthesia may be necessary for the shock delivery since patients experience the ICD shocks as painful and may feel uncomfortable in the phase when ventricular fibrillation is induced.

The implantation of a pectoral ICD step-by-step, and some examples of implanted ICD systems and stored events can be seen in **7.2–7.11**.

## Conclusion

Implantable defibrillators are highly developed devices and can easily be implanted in patients at risk of sudden death. However, cost effectiveness is also important and therefore further studies are needed to find the ideal patients for implantation. Prophylactic implantation seems to be the challenge of the future as we should prevent our patients from having to be resuscitated or die from ventricular fibrillation. On the other hand, quality of life is an important issue and new options should be investigated to treat heart failure more effectively, a condition which often leads to severe symptoms. Preventing sudden death is important but it is only part of what counts.

## References

1 Mirowski M, Reid PR, Mower MM, *et al.* (1980). Termination of malignant ventricular arrhythmias with an implanted automatic defibrillator in human beings. *N Engl J Med*, **303**:322–324.

2 Rosenquist M, Beyer T, Block M, *et al.* (1998). Adverse events with transvenous implantable cardioverter-defibrillators. *Circulation*, **98**: 663–670.

3 Priori SG, Aliot E, Blomstrom-Lundqvist C, *et al.* (2001). Task Force on sudden cardiac death of the European Society of Cardiology. *Europ Heart J*, **22**:1374–1450.

4 Gregoratos G, Abrahams J, Epstein A, *et al.* (2002). ACC/AHA/NASPE guideline update for implantation of cardiac pacemakers and antiarrhythmia devices. *Circulation*, **106**:2145–2161.

5 Priori SG, Aliot E, Blomstrom-Lundqvist C, *et al.* (2002). Task Force on sudden cardiac death, European Society of Cardiology. *Europace*, **4**:3–18.

6 Priori SG, Aliot E, Blomstrom-Lundqvist C, *et al.* (2003). Update of the guidelines on sudden cardiac death of the European Society of Cardiology. *Europ Heart J*, **24**:13–15.

**7.2** Tip of three common leads that can be connected to an implantable cardioverter-defibrillator. Top: Ventricular lead with passive fixation to be placed in the right ventricle in order to enable bipolar sensing and pacing and defibrillation via the shock coil which can be seen on the left side of the picture. Centre: Ventricular lead with active fixation (screw at the tip) with the same function as the above mentioned lead. Bottom: Shock coil only for defibrillation to be placed, for example, in the superior vena cava.

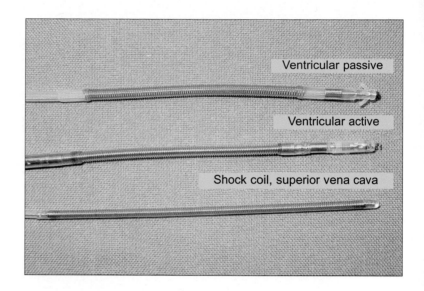

Ventricular passive

Ventricular active

Shock coil, superior vena cava

**7.3 (A, B)** Examples of abdominal implantable cardioverter-defibrillator devices and much smaller new devices which can be implanted subpectorally or even subcutaneously.

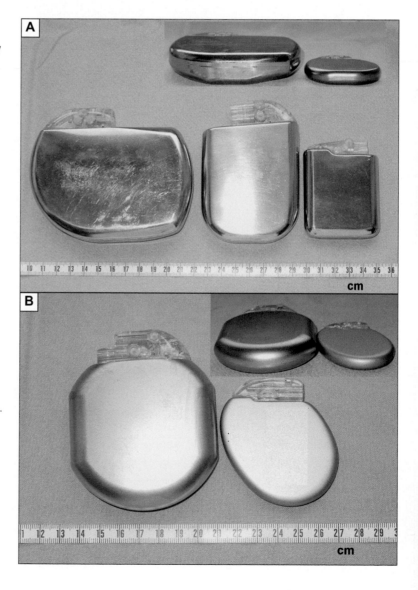

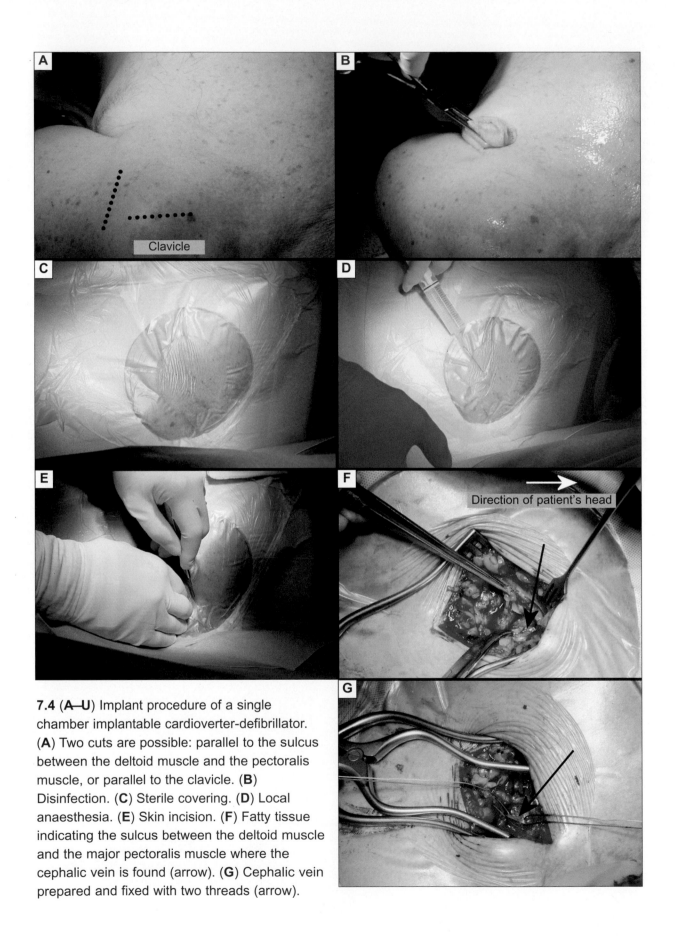

**7.4 (A–U)** Implant procedure of a single chamber implantable cardioverter-defibrillator. (**A**) Two cuts are possible: parallel to the sulcus between the deltoid muscle and the pectoralis muscle, or parallel to the clavicle. (**B**) Disinfection. (**C**) Sterile covering. (**D**) Local anaesthesia. (**E**) Skin incision. (**F**) Fatty tissue indicating the sulcus between the deltoid muscle and the major pectoralis muscle where the cephalic vein is found (arrow). (**G**) Cephalic vein prepared and fixed with two threads (arrow).

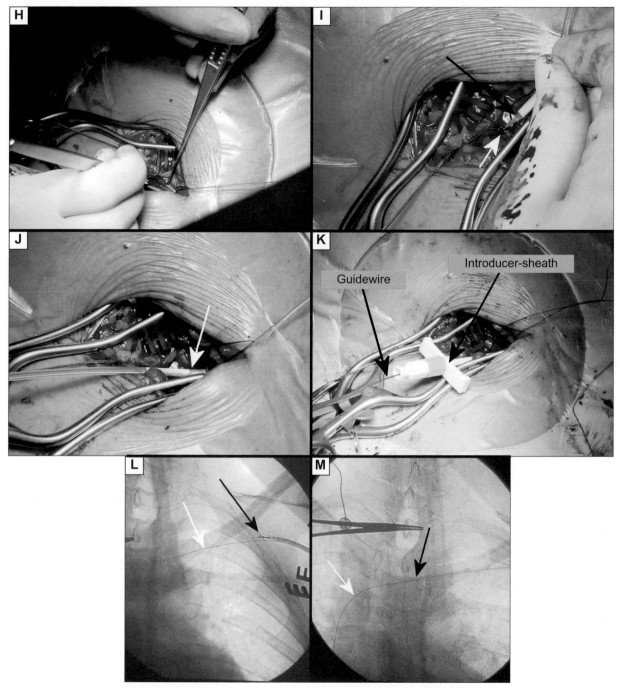

**7.4 (A–U)** Implant procedure of a single chamber implantable cardioverter-defibrillator (*continued*). (**H**) Incision of the cephalic vein held by a small forceps. (**I**) Opening of the vein (black arrow) with a little hook; the distal end of the vein is already ligated to prevent bleeding (white arrow). (**J**) Careful introduction of the lead into the vein, the beginning of the vessel is marked by the white arrow. To facilitate the introduction of the lead the distal suture may be pulled gently. (**K**) In case the lead does not advance properly into the subclavian vein because of valves or curves of the cephalic vein, a long soft guidewire may be inserted via the vein into the right atrium to indicate the right pathway. The introduction of a guiding sheath over the wire must be done under fluoroscopy to prevent kinking of the sheath or perforation of the vein. (**L**) Intraoperative fluoroscopy showing a guidewire advancing into the subclavian vein (white arrow), whereas the lead is stuck (black arrow). (**M**) Intraoperative fluoroscopy showing the guidewire in place (white arrow) and the tip of the introducer sheath in the subclavian vein (black arrow) without kinking.

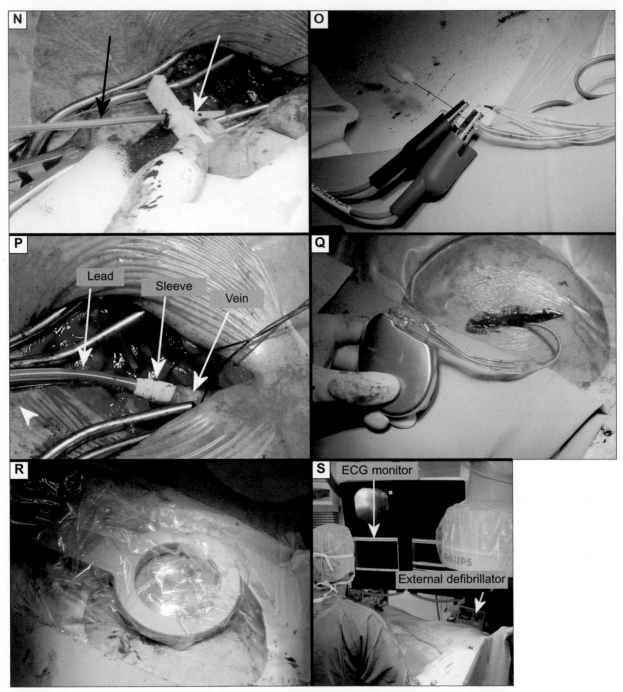

**7.4 (A–U)** Implant procedure of a single chamber implantable cardioverter-defibrillator (ICD) (*continued*). (**N**) Introduction of the lead (black arrow) into the sheath (white arrow). It is important to check for blood flow out of the sheath after removing the guidewire and the inner dilating part of the sheath, to avoid air aspiration. Sometimes tilting of the patient may be necessary. (**O**) After placing the lead in the right ventricle measurements of the intracardiac signals (e.g. R-wave), stimulation impedance, and pacing threshold have to be performed. (**P**) To fix the lead the sleeve is introduced into the cephalic vein and fixed with nonresorbable sutures. (**Q**) Thorough fixation of the lead in the device and testing for tightness of the screws (pulling on the lead) is required. (**R**) Intraoperative testing via the ICD *in situ* (in its subcutaneous or subpectoral pocket) and telemetry wand placed over the device. (**S**) Laboratory requirements: while inducing ventricular fibrillation for ICD testing an online electrocardiogram (ECG) and an external defibrillator in case of ICD failure have to be available.

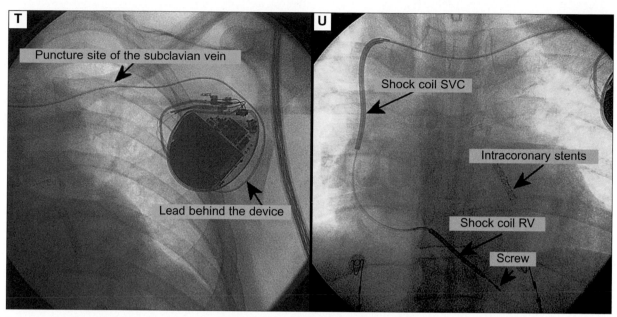

**7.4 (A–U)** Implant procedure of a single chamber implantable cardioverter-defibrillator (*continued*). (**T**) Final fluoroscopy check: the lead should not be damaged on its way into the subclavian vein and should be placed behind the device. (**U**) Final fluoroscopy check: the shock coils should be in the right place without kinking or twisting, and the tip of the lead should be screwed in properly. RV: right ventricle; SVC: superior vena cava.

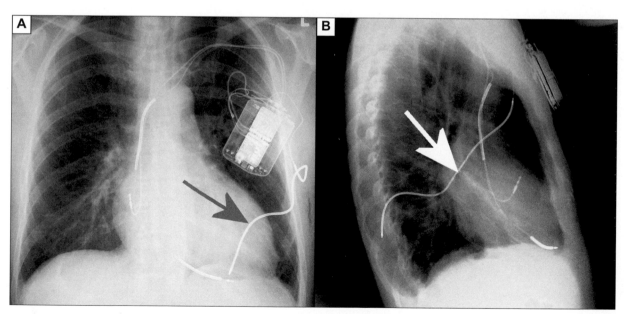

**7.5**   Chest X-ray (**A**: anteroposterior view; **B**: lateral view) after implantation of an implantable cardioverter-defibrillator (ICD) with an additional subcutaneous shock coil in a 62-year-old male patient who presented with ongoing ventricular tachycardia after syncope and several ICD discharges. The ICD was implanted 4 years before admission because of ventricular tachycardias and dilated cardiomyopathy. This time the patient experienced the onset of ventricular tachycardia but subsequent ICD shocks could not terminate the arrhythmia. The left ventricular ejection fraction decreased over time and at admission it was 20—25%. To solve the problem of ineffective ICD shocks with a rising defibrillation threshold an additional subcutaneous array electrode was implanted (arrow).

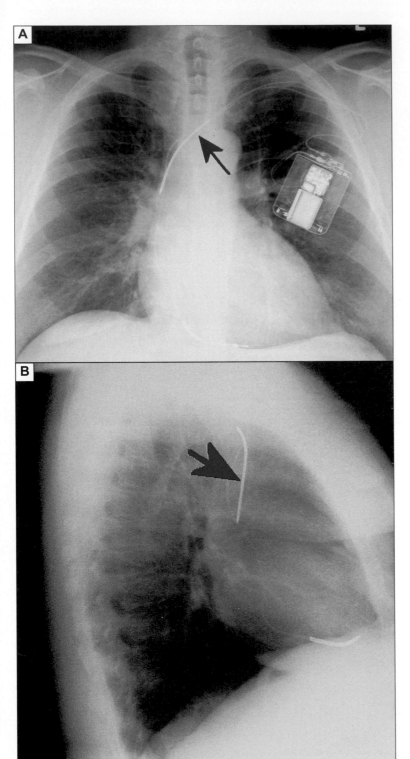

**7.6** Chest X-ray (**A**: anteroposterior view; **B**: lateral view) after implantation of an implantable cardioverter-defibrillator (ICD) in a 52-year-old obese male patient who presented with sustained ventricular tachycardia (cycle length 280 ms) which led to syncope and required cardioversion. The underlying heart disease was hypertensive cardiomyopathy with normal systolic left ventricular function. Although the tachycardia was inducible with programmed ventricular stimulation, a catheter ablation was not possible, because it required immediate cardioversion. Therefore, an ICD was implanted and the defibrillation threshold was sufficiently low after an additional superior vena cava lead (arrow) was implanted, and a high-energy device which could deliver 36 J shocks was implanted.

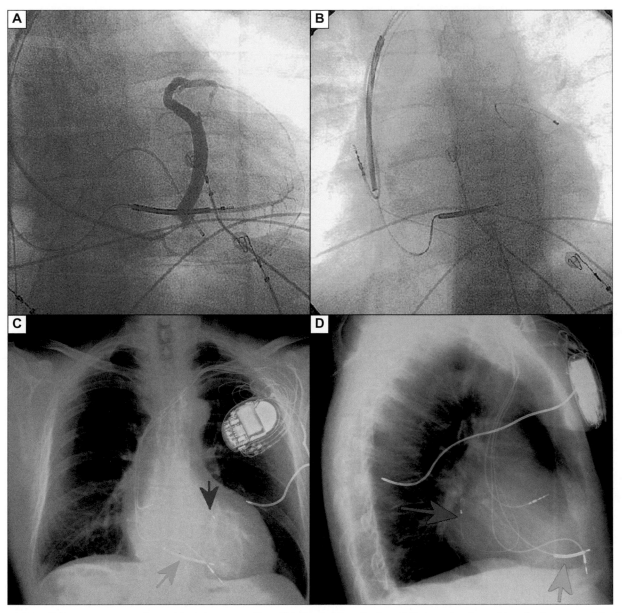

**7.7** Angiograms of the coronary sinus (**A**, intraoperative X-ray, right anterior oblique view) and lead placement in the coronary sinus (**B**, intraoperative X-ray, anteroposterior view). Chest X-ray (**C**, **D**) (anteroposterior and lateral view) after implantation of an implantable cardioverter-defibrillator (ICD) in a 44-year-old male patient with dilated cardiomyopathy and severely reduced systolic left ventricular ejection fraction (20%) who presented with an asymptomatic sustained ventricular tachycardia documented in a Holter electrocardiogram. Bundle branch re-entry was excluded by invasive electrophysiological investigation. One year earlier, the patient had undergone implantation of a biventricular pacemaker for resynchronization and now the pacemaker was replaced by an ICD. The coronary sinus electrode (stimulation of the left ventricle, red arrow) was kept *in situ*, as was the atrial lead. Only the defibrillation lead in the right ventricle had to be replaced (green arrow).

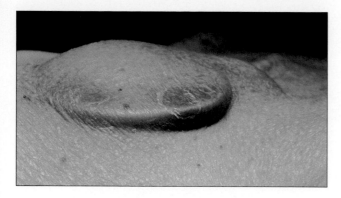

**7.8** Complications: detail of an infected device about to perforate.

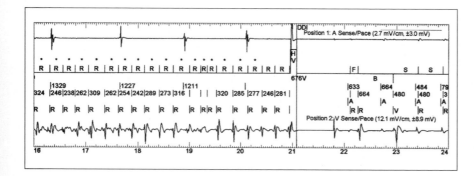

**7.9** ICD-derived intracardiac electrocardiogram (ECG), showing termination of ventricular fibrillation with DC shock. Upper intracardiac channel: atrial lead ECG; Lower intracardiac channel: ventricular ECG. A: atrial pacing; V: ventricular pacing; R: ventricular sensing; HV: shock delivery by ICD; ICD: implantable cardioverter-defibrillator.

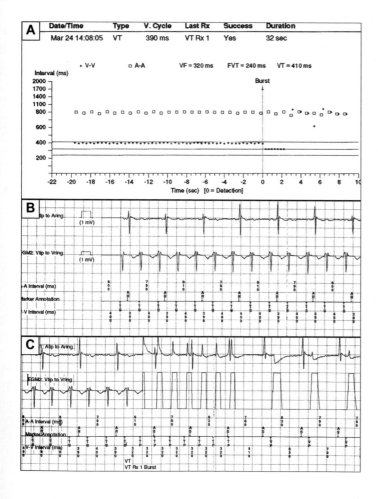

**7.10** (**A**) ICD-derived interval plot of a ventricular tachycardia and its termination. A: atrial sensing; V: ventricular sensing; VF: ventricular fibrillation; FVT: fast ventricular tachycardia; VT: ventricular tachycardia; Rx: therapy delivered by implantable cardioverter-defibrillator (ICD). (**B**) ICD-derived intracardiac electrocardiogram (ECG), showing detection of ventricular tachycardia. EGM: intracardiac ECG; A/V tip: atrial/ventricular lead tip EGM; A/V ring: atrial/ventricular ring EGM; AR: sensed atrial event within the refractory period; TS: tachycardia sensed event. (**C**) ICD-derived intracardiac ECG, showing termination of ventricular tachycardia with burst pacing and ongoing VAT pacing because of underlying total AV block. Channel annotation as in (**B**). AS: sensed atrial event; AR: sensed atrial event within the refractory period; VS: sensed ventricular event; VP: paced ventricular event; TS: tachycardia sensed event; Rx: therapy delivered by ICD.

**7.11 (A)** ICD-derived intracardiac ECG, showing inadequate detection of ventricular tachycardia in atrial tachycardia. Intracardiac ECG from top to bottom: atrial, ventricular, shock coil (far field). AS: sensed atrial event; VS: sensed ventricular event; VT: ventricular tachycardia event; VF: ventricular fibrillation event. **(B)** ICD-derived intracardiac ECG, inadequate burst pacing therapy in atrial tachycardia. Intracardiac ECG from top to bottom: atrial, ventricular, shock coil (far field). AS: sensed atrial event; VS: sensed ventricular event; VT: ventricular tachycardia event; VF: ventricular fibrillation event. **(C)** ICD-derived intracardiac ECG, showing inadequate cardioversion therapy in atrial tachycardia with induction of a nonsustained ventricular tachycardia and ongoing atrial tachycardia. Intracardiac ECG from top to bottom: atrial, ventricular, shock coil (far field). AS: sensed atrial event; ECG: electrocardiogram; ICD: implantable cardioverter-defibrillator; VS: sensed ventricular event; VT: ventricular tachycardia; VF: ventricular fibrillation.

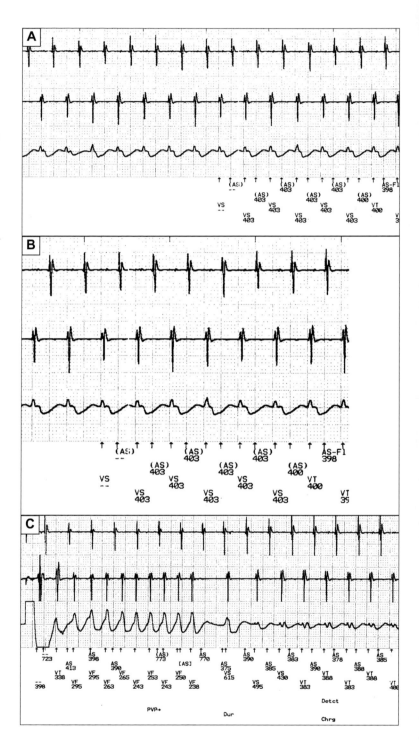

# Chapter 8

# Mitral Valvuloplasty

*Mario Togni, MD, and Bernhard Meier, MD*

## Introduction

Percutaneous mitral balloon valvuloplasty was introduced in 1984 by Inoue as an alternative to surgical mitral valve commissurotomy for the treatment of rheumatic mitral stenosis[1]. After two decades of experience with this technique it is clear that mitral balloon valvuloplasty is a safe and effective alternative to surgical repair in selected patients with mitral stenosis. Percutaneous mitral balloon valvuloplasty provides short-term palliation, as is the case with valvuloplasty for congenital aortic stenosis, and achieves also favourable mid-term results (follow-up data up to 10 years)[2, 3].

## Technical considerations

A variety of technical approaches may be used for percutaneous mitral balloon valvuloplasty. A transvenous, or antegrade, method is most commonly performed, with a trans-septal puncture used to gain access to the left atrium. Less often, a retrograde, transarterial approach is used to avoid the creation of a septal defect.

### Trans-septal puncture

Trans-septal catheterization is the first step of the procedure and is one of the most crucial. It is performed through the femoral vein. A Mullins sheath is advanced into the superior vena cava over a 0.035 inch guide wire. A Brockenbrough trans-septal needle is then advanced to the tip of the sheath. Both are slowly withdrawn as a unit, with the tip orientated in a 4 to 6 o'clock position relative to the needle stopcock position outside the body, which is in line with the direction of the needle tip in the heart. In patients with significant mitral stenosis there is distortion of the usual anatomy,

which usually requires that the needle and sheath be pointed more posteriorly. A manifold bank may be connected to the needle to allow flushing, contrast medium injection, and transducer attachment for continuous pressure observation.

As the needle and sheath are withdrawn, there are three pronounced movements of the sheath–needle combination toward the spine in the antero-posterior projection. The first movement is due to the passage of the sheath across the deflection of the superior vena cava with the right atrium; the second is due to movement along the bulging of the aorta and the right atrium; and the third is due to engagement of the fossa ovalis, upon which atrial pulsations are felt in the sheath. A pigtail catheter placed in the area of the aortic valve may be used to mark the anterior location of the aorta and to decrease the likelihood of inadvertent puncture of the aorta by an approach made too anteriorly.

The authors always confirm correct location of the sheath–needle combination by means of lateral fluoroscopy and dye marking of the point selected for puncture. While the needle is advanced to perform the puncture, it is attached to the manifold and small amounts of dye are injected into the septum (**8.1**). 'Tenting' of the septum indicates a good place for puncture (**8.2**). Once the position is correct, the needle is further advanced into the left atrium and on reaching the left atrium is checked with dye or through pressure monitoring to affirm successful completion of the puncture (**8.3**). The Mullins sheath is then advanced into the left atrium and the needle removed. A guide wire is advanced through the catheter into the left atrium. After trans-septal puncture a clinically irrelevant atrial septal defect may be noted (iatrogenic Lutembacher syndrome) (**8.4**). Complications of the trans-septal puncture include pericardial haemorrhage with cardiac tamponade and erroneous aortic puncture (**8.5**). Once access to the left atrium is established, a wire or balloon is passed across the mitral valve into the left ventricle (**8.6**). This may not be easily achieved, especially with low trans-septal punctures, and an indirect approach with looping of the balloon over the pigtail wire in the left atrium has to then be performed (**8.7**).

Two types of balloon approaches are used for percutaneous mitral balloon valvuloplasty. With the double balloon method, two trans-septal punctures are performed and two balloon catheters are advanced simultaneously across the mitral valve into the left ventricle. To avoid the second trans-septal puncture, the two wires may be advanced through the same hole using an exchange catheter (**8.8**) or special valvuloplasty balloons can be used. For example, Bifoil or Trefoil balloons with two or three balloons, respectively, side by side on a single shaft (**8.9**), or a balloon encompassing the wire only at the tip with a standard balloon inserted on the same wire behind it. These techniques have been largely abandoned due to the high incidence of severe mitral regurgitation and a significant risk of ventricular perforation by the balloon tip(s) during systole with the balloon(s) fixed in the mitral valve. The Inoue balloon allows passage into the left ventricle with a rounded tip avoiding small gaps between the chordae. It can easily be fixed in the stenotic valve when inflating the distal part only, to pull the balloon back into the valve and it affords progressive diameter dilatation by increasing the filling volume (**8.6**, **8.10–8.14**). A stepwise dilatation technique is advantageous to minimize the risk of mitral valve rupture and regurgitation.

## Assessment of result

Serial haemodynamic measurements are used to evaluate the result achieved with percutaneous mitral balloon valvuloplasty. An immediate improvement in left atrial mean pressure and reduction of the transmitral gradient should be seen, with a gradual decrease in pulmonary artery pressure and an increase in cardiac output. Criteria for termination of the procedure include: (1) drop of the mitral valve pressure gradient to a few mmHg (**8.12**, **8.13**); (2) a mitral valve area $>1$ cm$^2$/m$^2$ body surface area; (3) complete opening of at least one commissure if echocardiography is available during the procedure; or (4) new or increased mitral regurgitation by left ventriculography (**8.14**), increase of the V-wave of the left atrial pressure (**8.13**), or Doppler echocardiography.

## Immediate results

In a series of 2538 patients with mitral stenosis treated with mitral balloon valvuloplasty, Iung and coworkers report a decrease of mean left atrial pressure from $22\pm7$ mmHg to $13\pm5$ mmHg, with an increase of valve area from $1.0\pm0.2$ cm$^2$ to $1.92\pm0.31$ cm$^2$.[4] In 30 cases (1.3%) the procedure was not completed because of complications that occurred before percutaneous mitral balloon valvuloplasty (haemopericardium or embolism) or due to technical failure (inability to puncture or to cross the interatrial septum or to position the balloon correctly across the mitral valve). Major adverse events reported in the series include in-hospital death in 11 patients (0.4%), embolism with sequelae in 9 (0.4%), and severe mitral regurgitation in 95 (3.8%).

**8.1** Trans-septal puncture step 1 (lateral view). Injection of contrast medium into the interatrial septum depicts that the approach is too parallel or tangential to the septum. A clockwise rotation of the needle tip to the right side of the screen is required for successful passage into the left atrium. LV: left ventricle; LA: left atrium; RA: right atrium.

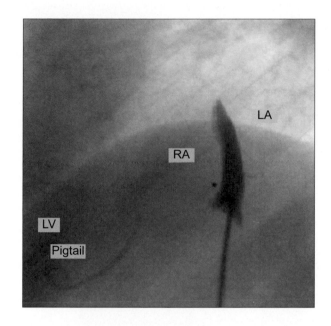

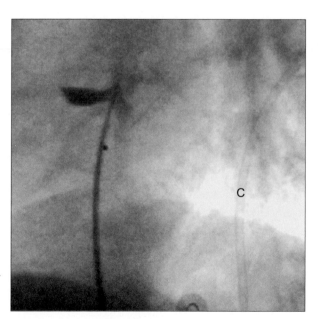

**8.2** Trans-septal puncture step 2 (lateral view). Tenting of the septum while advancing the needle indicates the correct direction of the needle. C: catheter in descending aorta.

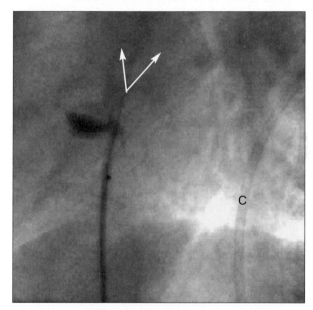

**8.3** Trans-septal puncture step 3 (lateral view). Successful perforation of the septum. Injection of dye into the left atrium (arrows) can confirm correct positioning. C: catheter in descending aorta.

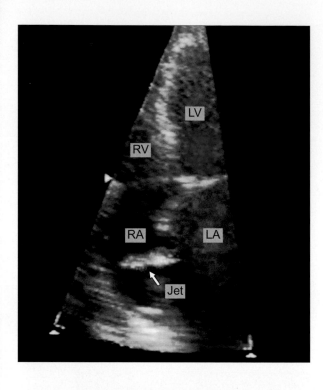

**8.4** Atrial septal defect after trans-septal puncture. Transthoracic echocardiography, four chamber view. Jet originating in the left atrium is directed into the right atrium. LV: left ventricle; RV: right ventricle; LA: left atrium; RA: right atrium.

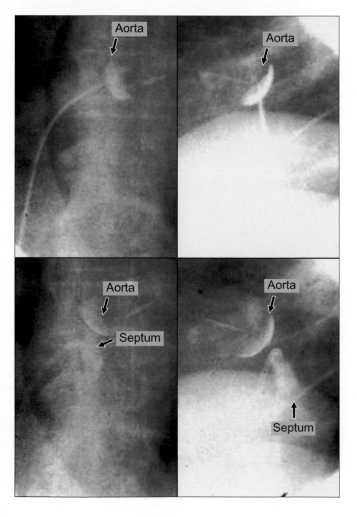

**8.5** Inadvertent aortic puncture. Left panels: postero-anterior projection. Right panels: corresponding lateral projection. Upper panels: Inadvertent puncture of the ascending aorta with injection of dye into the posterior aortic wall. Lower panels: Correct puncture of the interatrial septum with introduction of a catheter into the left atrium. The lateral projection distinguishes much better between aorta and interatrial septum than the postero-anterior projection.

**8.6** Schematic diagram of the Inoue procedure of percutaneous mitral valvuloplasty. (1) Trans-septal access to the left atrium. (2) Advancement of the balloon through the mitral valve. (3, 4) Inflation of the balloon.

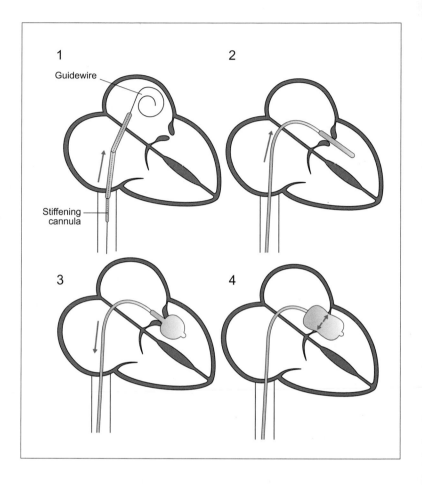

**8.7** Indirect advancement of a balloon with counterclockwise looping of the balloon over the pigtail introducer wire in the left atrium. This manoeuvre may become necessary in cases of a low puncture of the interatrial septum rendering the direct approach impossible. Advancement of the Inoue balloon is always performed with slight inflation of the distal end to avoid passage through a small mesh gap between the chordae tendinae, which would then rupture during balloon inflation and potentially cause severe mitral regurgitation.

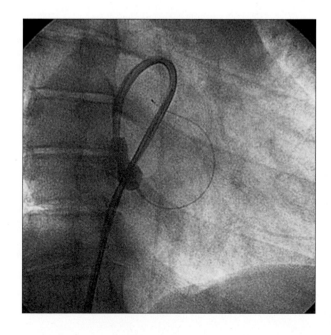

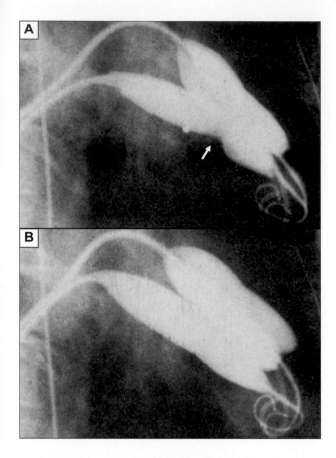

**8.8** Double balloon percutaneous mitral valvuloplasty using two separate balloons. In this case, a single and a Bifoil balloon were inserted through the same trans-septal hole on two separate guidewires. (**A**) Shows the indentation by the mitral valve (arrow) before full opening (**B**).

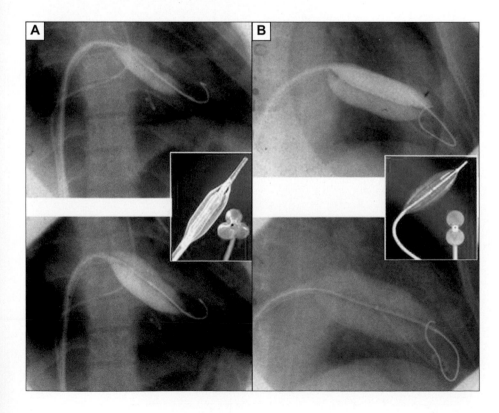

**8.9** Trefoil (**A**, 3 × 15 mm) and Bifoil (**B**, 2 × 19 mm) mitral balloon valvuloplasty through a 16 French trans-septal sheath, before (upper panels) and after (lower panels) full inflation. The inserts depict the respective balloons in frontal and orthogonal views.

**8.10** Inoue balloon percutaneous mitral commissurotomy technique (see also **8.6**). After trans-septal puncture and introduction of a coiled guide wire (pigtail wire) into the left atrium, the Inoue balloon is advanced into the left ventricle. After inflation of the distal portion of the balloon in the fundus of the left ventricle (**A**) it is pulled back and anchored at the mitral valve. Subsequently, the proximal and middle portions of the balloon are filled (**B**). At full inflation the waist of the balloon in its mid-portion has disappeared as a sign of successful comissurotomy (**C**).

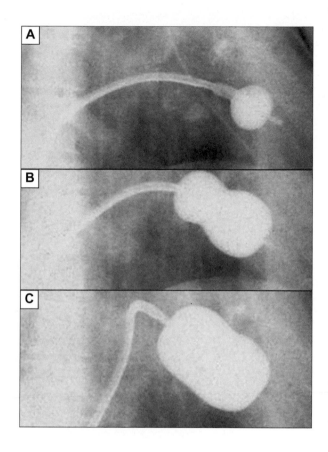

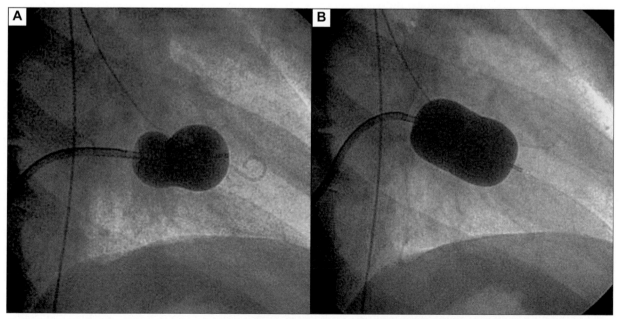

**8.11** The waist diameter can be volume controlled from 24 mm (**A**) to 30 mm (**B**) with the most commonly used Inoue balloon size.

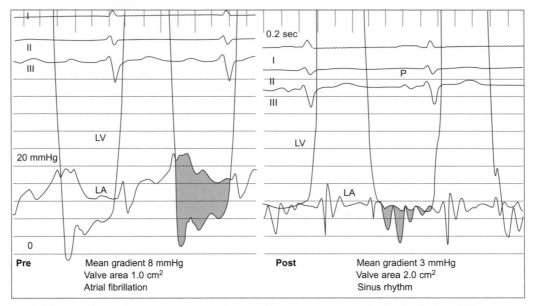

**8.12** Haemodynamic assessment of percutaneous mitral valvuloplasty in a 50-year-old patient with rheumatic mitral stenosis. Before the procedure the left atrial pressures as well as the transmitral pressure gradient are elevated. The calculated mitral valve area is 1.0 cm². Valvuloplasty results in a decrease of both left atrial pressures and transmitral pressure gradient to values in the normal range. The post-procedure mitral valve area rises to 2.0 cm² and the patient was electrically converted to sinus rhythm at the end of the procedure. LA: left atrium; LV: left ventricle; P: P-wave.

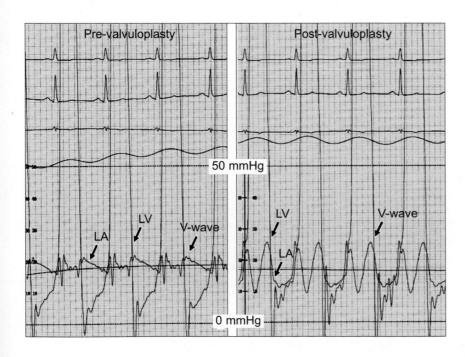

**8.13** Haemodynamic measurements in a case of Inoue mitral balloon valvuloplasty. The gradient is again abolished without significant increase of the left atrial V-wave. The left atrial curve of the left panel is in fact a pulmonary wedge pressure. This explains the less phasic and somewhat delayed excursions compared with the left atrial curve of the right panel measured in the left atrium through the central lumen of the Inoue balloon. LA: left atrium; LV: left ventricle.

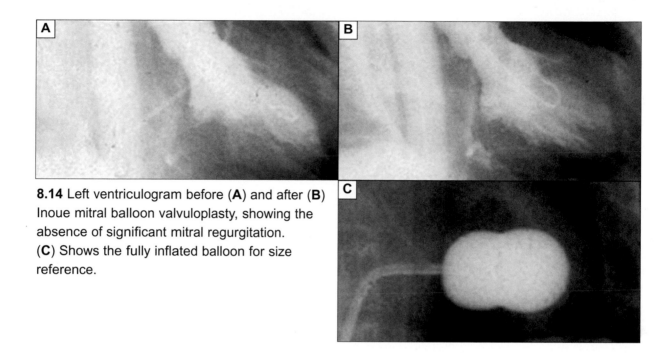

**8.14** Left ventriculogram before (**A**) and after (**B**) Inoue mitral balloon valvuloplasty, showing the absence of significant mitral regurgitation. (**C**) Shows the fully inflated balloon for size reference.

## Mid-term and long-term follow-up

Follow-up 7–10 years after percutaneous mitral balloon valvuloplasty in five series including more than 2500 patients, show a survival rate of 83–95%[2, 5–8]. Freedom from operation is reported in 61–84%, with a functional New York Heart Association class I or II occurring in 52–75% of patients. These data are encouraging and show that valvuloplasty is at least comparable to surgical commissurotomy with regards to mid-term follow-up[9].

## Conclusion

The majority of mitral valvuloplasty procedures are performed in developing countries, where rheumatic heart disease is endemic. There, mitral valvuloplasty has an important place in the treatment of mitral stenosis and is being used as an alternative to definitive surgical repair or replacement in selected patients with symptomatic mitral stenosis. The good results obtained with this technique have resulted in mitral valvuloplasty virtually replacing surgical commissurotomy in young patients and it should also be tried before surgery in the elderly with mitral stenosis.

## References

1 Inoue K, Owaki T, Nakamura T, *et al.* (1984). Clinical application of transvenous mitral commissurotomy by a new balloon catheter. *J Thorac Surg*, **87**:394–402.

2 Iung B, Garbarz E, Michaud P, *et al.* (1999). Late results of percutaneous mitral commissurotomy in a series of 1024 patients: analysis of late clinical deterioration: frequency, anatomic findings, and predictive factors. *Circulation*, **99**:3272–3278.

3 Palacious IF, Tuzcu ME, Weyman AE, *et al.* (1995). Clinical follow-up of patients undergoing percutaneous mitral balloon valvotomy. *Circulation*, **91**:671–676.

4 Iung B, Cormier B, Ducimetiere P, *et al.* (1996). Immediate results of percutaneous mitral commissurotomy. *Circulation*, **94**:2124–2130.

5 Hernandez R, Banuelos C, Alfonso F, *et al.* (1999). Long-term clinical and echocardiographic follow-up after percutaneous mitral valvuloplasty with the Inoue balloon. *Circulation*, **99**:1580–1586.

6 Meneveau N, Schiele F, Seronde MF, *et al.* (1998). Predictors of event-free survival after percutaneous mitral commissurotomy. *Heart*, **80**:359–364.

7 Orrange SE, Kawanishi Lopez BM, Curry SM, *et al.* (1997). Actuarial outcome after catheter balloon commissurotomy in patients with mitral stenosis. *Circulation*, **95**:382–389.

8 Stefanadis C, Stratos C, Lambrou S, *et al.* (1998). Retrograde nontrans-septal balloon mitral valvuloplasty: immediate results and intermediate long-term outcome in 441 cases: a multi-center experience. *J Am Coll Cardiol*, **32**:1009–1016.

9 Reyes VP, Raju BS, Wynne J, *et al.* (1994). Percutaneous balloon valvuloplasty compared with open surgical commissurotomy for mitral stenosis. *N Engl J Med*, **331**:961–967.

# Chapter 9

# Percutaneous Left Ventricular Assist Device

*Sandy Watson, RN, BN, and Bernhard Meier, MD*

## Introduction

Percutaneous left ventricular assistance was first performed on dogs in 1959[1], and on humans a few years later[2]. A roller pump took blood from the left atrium through a trans-septal catheter and pumped it into the descending aorta (**9.1**). The system was plagued by the technical limitations of the time, the thrombogenicity of the tubing being the primary problem. The idea was taken up again in the late 1980s in shock patients undergoing angioplasty, but the results were mixed[3]. Technology had developed to such an extent, however, that a number of patients (in a different setting) were supported for up to 10 days on a percutaneous left ventricular assistance device[4].

Over 40 years after the first attempt, only the TandemHeart (Cardiac Assist Inc, Pittsburgh, USA), is available for clinical use. Twenty-four patients have been treated with the TandemHeart over the past few years at the authors' institution, and more than 200 worldwide at the end of 2003. The advantage of the TandemHeart system is that it can be inserted in the cardiac catheterization laboratory setting, on awake patients, under local anaesthesia.

The TandemHeart is a centrifugal pump (max 7200 revolutions per minute [RPM]) that has a low blood–surface contact area. This reduces the probability of haemolysis and of thromboembolism. The pump itself is somewhat smaller than a clenched fist (**9.2**), and is practically silent while in operation. It provides a continuous, rather than pulsatile flow.

The TandemHeart harvests blood from the left atrium through a 21 French trans-septal catheter, and pumps it into the distal aorta via one or two 12, 15, or 17 French arterial cannulae (**9.3**). The insertion can be accomplished in about 20 minutes, and both the trans-septal and the arterial cannulae can be placed on the same side of the patient's groin (**9.4**), sparing the other side for additional interventions, such as coronary angioplasty.

## Indications

There are four types of patients who can benefit from percutaneous assist devices. The first is acute heart failure patients. A left ventricular assist device can give temporary support as a bridge to recovery[6] or to some other type of therapy, such as transplantation. The positioning of the cannulae in the groin precludes mobilization while the system is in place. This means that it can only be used as a temporary bridge to some other form of therapy. The longest that a TandemHeart has been in place in a patient is 23 days. If recovery is not imminent within the first 10 days, surgical placement of a more permanent device, which allows for patient ambulation, should be considered.

The second group of potential recipients is that of coronary artery disease patients with severely impaired left ventricular function. A patient in cardiogenic shock can have angioplasty performed irrespective of ventricular function, and recovery of myocardial function may be assisted in the days following revascularization if a left ventricular assist device is implanted in conjunction with angioplasty[7].

The third patient type who may benefit from the insertion of a left ventricular assist device are those undergoing elective high-risk procedures. The dilation of a left main lesion or a last remaining vessel can be performed under the protection of a left ventricular assist device[8]. Since the implantation of an assist device can ensure adequate blood flow even in the case of a prolonged vessel occlusion, the risk of mortality related to angioplasty can be reduced.

The fourth is the patient undergoing closed heart cardiac surgery under TandemHeart support.

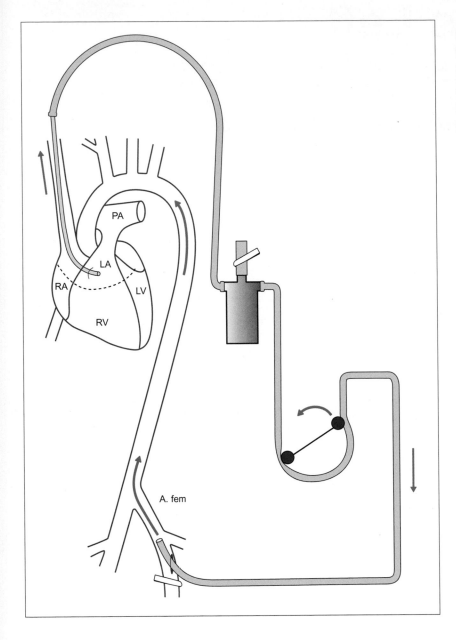

**9.1** Schematic of a roller pump left atrium to femoral artery bypass. The reservoir is fed only by gravity from the left atrium. A. fem: femoral artery; LA: left atrium; LV: left ventricle; PA: pulmonary artery; RA: right atrium; RV: right ventricle. (Courtesy of Hall *et al.*[5])

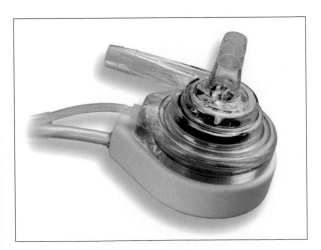

**9.2** TandemHeart pump.

**9.3** Venous sheath placed trans-septally in the left atrium and connected via the pump on the right thigh, with arterial catheters in the right and left iliac arteries. Commonly only one arterial catheter is used.

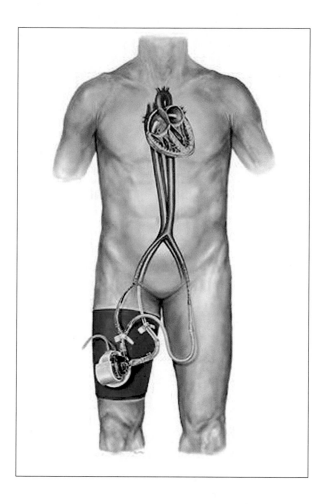

**9.4** A patient supported by the TandemHeart can be awake including during implantation and removal. The patient is fairly comfortable but cannot be mobilized. The insert shows the catheters in the right groin area.

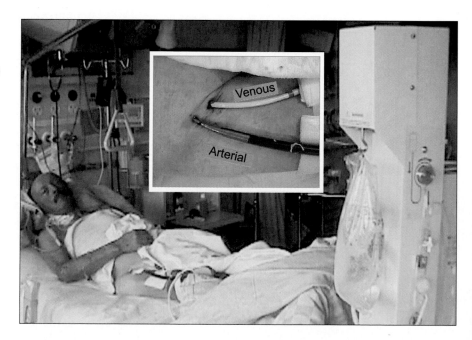

## System components

The TandemHeart pump is comprised of two chambers (**9.5**). The upper chamber houses the impellor and has the inflow and outflow conduits, and the lower chamber contains the electromagnetic drive system for the impellor, and a feedback mechanism to the controller, which can estimate the amount of blood that is being pumped. The lower chamber is infused with a heparinized solution (either distilled water or saline) which serves as a hydrodynamic bearing, as a coolant, and as an anticoagulant at the point of contact between the pump and blood. The impellor actually rests in this solution, meaning that there is no true contact between the impellor and the pump's lower housing.

The controller is a free-standing unit that has a touch-sensitive display panel (**9.6**). The panel displays the RPM at which the pump is functioning, and the approximate volume of blood that it pumped per minute. Should an alarm be triggered, the source of the alarm is displayed in the upper, right hand corner. More details about the pump's functioning will be displayed when the system data area in the lower right of the screen is pressed. The controller's display screen is made up of two identical sections, an upper and a lower. It normally runs on the upper part, but if this should fail, the clapper is folded up and the lower section will take over control of the pump.

Two cannulae are used with the TandemHeart system (**9.7**). The trans-septal cannula has been developed by Cardiac Assist to pass through the fossa ovalis and rest in the left atrium. The distal end has a large hole, and in the last few centimetres of the cannula there are side holes to facilitate the harvesting of blood. There is a radiopaque ring on the obturator just proximal to the side holes in the cannula, which helps with accurate positioning. There are also markers on the cannula's proximal shaft to verify its depth in the patient, which are helpful in ensuring that the trans-septal catheter remains in the correct position while the patient is being cared for in the intensive care unit.

Arterial cannulae of varying sizes can be used. Angiography of the pelvic arteries helps to select the appropriate size of the arterial cannula (**9.8**). While the 17 French catheter provides the best flow, it may cause leg ischaemia especially in smaller patients or in patients with peripheral vascular disease. A 15 French or smaller catheter may be preferable in these cases. With these smaller gauge catheters the flow will be reduced. A second cannula can be placed in the opposite groin, and connected with a 'Y' piece provided with the set (**9.3**). Likewise, a side arm of the arterial tube may be connected to a 6–8 French sheath inserted antegradely into the superficial femoral artery, to improve leg perfusion.

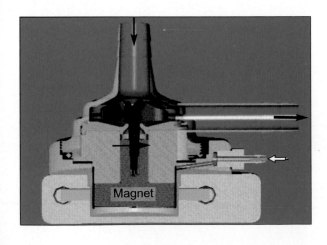

**9.5** Cut-away diagram of the TandemHeart pump, showing the upper and the lower chambers. In the upper chamber, a turbine (impellor) propels the blood entering through the vertical tube out the horizontal tube. In the lower chamber, the magnetic axle is electrically rotated. Lubrification is assured with heparinized flush through a side port (white arrow) that becomes mixed with the blood, heparinizing the patient to a certain degree.

**9.6** The TandemHeart controller. The display indicates revolutions per minute (RPM) and an estimate of the pumped blood volume per minute.

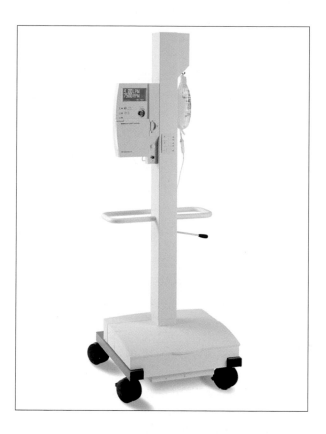

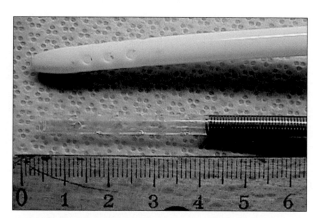

**9.7** Venous 21 French trans-septal and 15 French arterial cannulae used with the TandemHeart system. The ruler indicates cm.

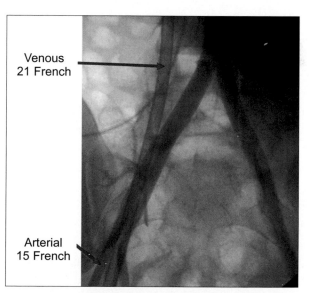

**9.8** Arterial and venous cannulae in place in a 22-year-old patient with end-stage cardiomyopathy and fairly small iliac arteries. A 15 French arterial cannula was selected.

## Implantation technique

The fossa ovalis of the interatrial septum is reached with the use of a standard Mullins trans-septal catheter inserted preferably via the right femoral vein (see Chapter 8). A Brockenbrough needle is advanced into the left atrium. Staining of the septum helps to identify the place of trans-septal puncture (**9.9**). A wire is passed through the trans-septal catheter into the left atrium (**9.10**). The preferred wire for this is the pigtail wire used for mitral valvuloplasty with an Inoue balloon (Toray Europe, Ltd). Once the wire is in place, the needle and the sheath are removed and replaced by the two-stage, trans-septal dilator. When this has been passed through the fossa ovalis it is replaced by the 21 French trans-septal cannula (**9.11**). The wire is removed, and the cannula is double-clamped. The cannula's positioning is checked by fluoroscopy (**9.11, 9.12**).

The artery is then accessed and the arterial cannula is inserted. Once the arterial cannula has been placed, it should also be double-clamped, awaiting connection to the pump.

During the time of cannula insertion, the controller and the infusion line are prepared. The controller is plugged into the power outlet and switched on. A 1 litre bag of sterile water or saline has 90,000 units of heparin added to it, and this is hung on the hook of the controller, next to the display panel. The bag is then punctured with the spike of the provided infusion line. A three-way stopcock, then the transducer, and then the bacterial filter are connected to this. A large syringe is attached to the third port of the three-way stopcock, and is filled with heparinized water drawn from the bag. The infusion line can then be threaded through the tiny roller pump at the back of the controller. The body of the transducer is slotted into the holder underneath this, and the transducer connector is plugged into the adjacent port.

The pump itself is connected to the controller by a double line. The larger component is the drive cable, and the other carries the heparinized water to the pump. Both components are connected to their respective ports on the controller. The syringe full of infusate is used to fill the connecting line and the pump with heparinized water. The pump is held upright during the flushing, and it is given the occasional knock to dispel air bubbles.

Plastic tubing is provided in a set. It is cut into short lengths to connect the pump to the cannulae. The venous cannula is connected first, and the clamps loosened to allow the connecting tubing and the pump to be filled with blood. The arterial cannula is then connected, and the system is purged of air. The clamps are removed completely, and the pump is turned on, initially at slow speed to make sure that residual air in the system goes to the legs and does not reach the visceral vessels, let alone the aortic arch.

The position of the trans-septal cannula should be checked. If in doubt, a blood sample from the system's side connector can be checked for its oxygen content. Finally, both cannulae are sutured to the patient's skin. Plastic loop-clamps are fastened using the gun provided to give added security to the connections. The pump itself can then be clicked into the holster, and the holster connected to the rubber sheet that is wrapped around the patient's thigh.

## Monitoring

The patient is confined to the intensive care unit for the duration of the TandemHeart's support. Generous filling of the patient's vascular system is recommended. If deemed necessary, this can be monitored with a Swan Ganz catheter. In addition to routine checks of intensive care patients, hourly readings of the pump's speed and output are recorded. Free plasma haemoglobin is measured daily in addition to the normal blood values to monitor haemolysis. It is often unnecessary to give the patient additional anticoagulation, as the amount of heparin provided by the infusion (about 900 U/hour) maintains the patient's activated clotting time at the recommended 270 seconds.

Extra care must be given when the patient is washed, as it is possible that the trans-septal cannula is displaced if the patient is not rolled correctly. The upper body must be turned at the same time as the lower. Twisting of the body can result in the distal end of the trans-septal cannula slipping backwards through the fossa ovalis. If this occurs, the colour of the blood in the system will noticeably darken. Usually this means that a number of side holes are now in the right atrium, and the cannula needs to be repositioned by pushing it at the proximal end. A fully dislocated cannula, however, requires total repositioning or replacement.

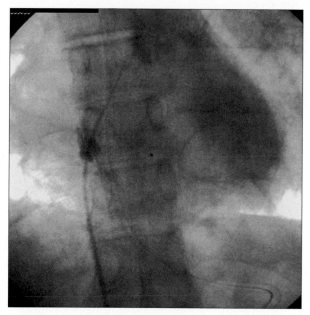

**9.9** The Brockenbrough needle punctures the fossa ovalis, rendered radiopaque with contrast staining.

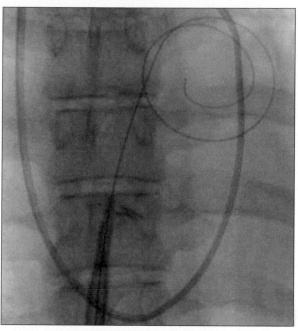

**9.10** A wire positioned in the left atrium. Commonly, the pigtail-type wire (part of the Inoue valvuloplasty set) is employed.

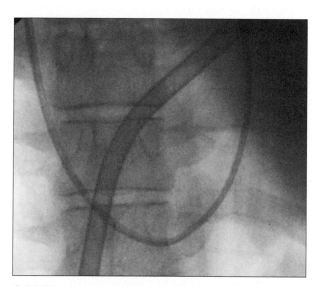

**9.11** The trans-septal cannula in position.

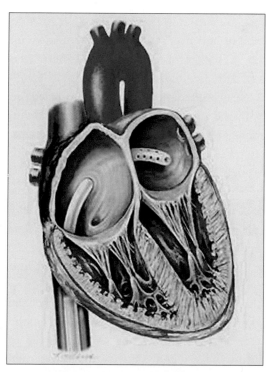

**9.12** Diagram of the ideal position of the trans-septal cannula.

## Weaning and explantation

The patient's progress can be assessed by turning down the speed of the TandemHeart to the minimum while monitoring the patient's cardiac function. When it has been determined that the system can be removed, a period of weaning is often instigated. This can go for a number of hours, or a day, depending on the patient's condition and how long the device has been in place.

Explantation can be performed at the bedside with manual compression in most cases. The sutures are cut and the pump is stopped. The tubing between the pump and the cannulae are clamped, and the cannulae are pulled out under manual pressure, as with any cannula removal. Owing to the large diameter of the arterial cannula, digital compression should be maintained for 1 hour and then a compression device should be left in place for about 6 hours. Surgical removal may be warranted if the patient is restless, the blood pressure is high, or anticoagulation cannot be interrupted for a few hours.

## Case report

A 55-year-old male patient was flown in by helicopter in cardiogenic shock. He had had a bland cardiac history up until a few months prior to admission, when he experienced atypical chest pain. His cardiologist performed a treadmill exercise test and an echocardiogram, which produced no abnormal results. In the weeks before admission, however, he began to experience increased dyspnoea during the night. This culminated in severe nocturnal shortness of breath with radiating pain through his left arm. He was admitted to a local hospital, where an echocardiogram showed an ejection fraction of <20%. A chest computer tomography (CT) scan showed massive pleural effusion and cardiomegaly. He was in atrial fibrillation, which was treated with amiodarone. As his condition continued to worsen, he was intubated and transferred to the authors' centre.

Angiography showed only a thrombotic occlusion of the patient's first diagonal branch, which was dilated and the thrombus aspirated. His ejection fraction was confirmed to be 20% with diffuse hypo- and akinesia. A myocardial biopsy was taken from the patient's right ventricular septum in an attempt to determine the cause of his cardiomyopathy. An intra-aortic balloon pump was inserted and vasopressors and intravenous heparin given.

The patient continued to be haemodynamically unstable, and the decision was made to replace the balloon pump with a TandemHeart. The patient was transported, still intubated, to the cardiac catheterization laboratory. Both groins were disinfected and the patient was draped.

The femoral vein was punctured in the right groin and the trans-septal cannula was inserted, using the technique described previously. Using a normal exchange wire, the 17 French arterial cannula was inserted. The TandemHeart was primed and connected without difficulty. The initial speed was 7500 RPM (approx 4 l/min). The TandemHeart pump was functioning within 10 min of the intra-aortic balloon pump being turned off.

The patient was returned to the intensive care unit for monitoring. Over the next few days his condition slowly improved, and the TandemHeart's speed could be reduced to 5200 RPM. The ejection fraction remained around 20% by echogardiographical estimation. The patient continued to experience intermittent atrial fibrillation; however, the urine output picked up, and the pleural effusion corrected itself completely on the right side, with some improvement on the left. The TandemHeart was removed on the fourth day, and the patient was extubated a day later. The biopsy samples were histologically normal, with no infectious infiltrates.

Three days after removal of the TandemHeart, only a very minor left to right shunt was echographically evident at the level of the atrial septum. This had completely resolved 10 days after removal. On the eighth day after admission, the patient was transferred to a normal ward, and he left the hospital a day later. His ejection fraction had improved to 40%. He was discharged under oral anticoagulation due to a sustained atrial flutter (which was successfully electroconverted at a later date); enalapril, diuretics, an aldosterone antagonist, beta-blocker, and amiodarone were also prescribed. The patient attended the hospital's rehabilitation programme and reports for regular follow-ups at the heart failure clinic.

## Conclusion

Ventricular assist devices have traditionally been implanted surgically, and only in cases of end-stage cardiac failure. Implantation of a percutaneous ventricular assist device is within the technical capabilities of most interventional cardiac catheterization laboratories. The amount of preparation time is minimal, and the insertion of the device cannulae can readily be combined with a diagnostic cardiac catheterization or a percutaneous revascularization procedure.

In contrast to the borderline effect of the intra-aortic balloon pump, the left ventricle is definitely unloaded by the TandemHeart, and ventricular, pulmonary, and atrial filling pressures are reduced. The aortic pressure printout without and then with the TandemHeart in action is shown (**9.13**). Cardiac output is improved, and organ perfusion is maintained irrespective of left ventricular function. When angioplasty is performed under TandemHeart support (**9.14**), an adequate arterial pressure is maintained throughout the procedure.

The system, however, relies on adequate right heart function (necessitating a regular cardiac rhythm) to maintain blood oxygenation levels. Some attempts have been made to couple the TandemHeart with an oxygenation system, but the pump's output pressure is inadequate, so right heart failure remains a contraindication for TandemHeart placement.

There are several studies in progress designed to determine under which situations implantation of a percutaneous left ventricular assist device is beneficial, and it appears likely that this device will find a niche in contemporary interventional cardiology.

**9.13** Aortic pressure without, and with (Pump on) the TandemHeart during balloon inflation.

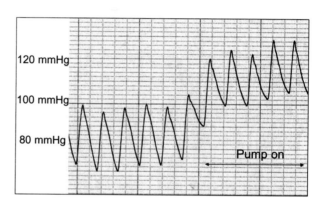

**9.14** Arterial pressure maintained at about 100 mmHg in a patient on TandemHeart support during angioplasty. Note the disappearance of the phasic signal after balloon inflation, proving that the left ventricle does no longer contribute to the cardiac output and the aortic valve stays closed. The insert shows the aortic flow before balloon inflation. There is a short antegrade flow (upward peak) corresponding to the opening of the aortic valve, followed by a long retrograde flow from the pump, assuring mainly the cardiac output.

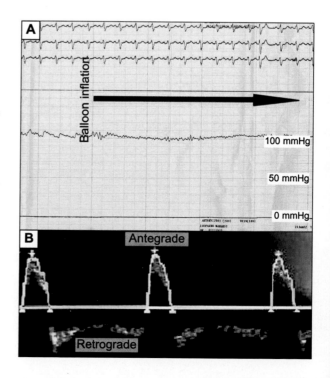

## References

1 Salisbury PF, Bor N, Levin RY, Rieben PA (1959). Effects of partial and total heart–lung bypass on the heart. *J App Physiol*, **14**: 458–463.

2 Senning A, Dennis C, Hall DP, Moreno JR (1962). Left atrial cannulation without thoracotomy for total left heart bypass. *Acta Chir Scand*, **123**:267–279.

3 Rose DM, Connolly M, Cunningham JN, Spencer FC (1989). Technique and results with a roller pump left and right heart assist device. *Ann Thorac Surg*, **47**:124–129.

4 Babic UU, Grujicic SN, Djurisic Z, Vucinic M (1988). Nonsurgical left atrial aortic bypass. *Lancet*, **2**:1430–1431.

5 Hall DP, Moreno JR, Dennis C, Senning A (1962). An experimental study of prolonged left heart bypass without thoracotomy. *Ann Surg*, **156**:190–196.

6 Westaby S, Katsumata T, Pigott D, Jin XY, Saatvedt K, Horton M, Clark RE (2000). Mechanical bridge to recovery in fulminant myocarditis. *Ann Thorac Surg*, **70**:278–283.

7 Thiele H, Lauer B, Hambrecht R, Boudriot E, Cohen H, Schuler G (2001). Reversal of cardiogenic shock by percutaneous left atrial-to-femoral arterial bypass assistance. *Circulation*, **104**:2917–2922.

8 Vranckx P, Foley DP, de Feijter PJ, Smits P, Serruys PW (2003). Clinical introduction of the TandemHeart, a percutaneous left ventricular assist device, for circulatory support during high-risk percutaneous coronary interventions. *Int J Cardiovasc Intervent*, **5**:35–39.

# Index